Multiple-choice Questions in Otolaryngology
with explanatory answers

Multiple-choice Questions in Otolaryngology
with explanatory answers

Ramindar S. Dhillon, FRCS (Eng)
James W. Fairley, FRCS (Eng)

Ferens Institute of Otolaryngology
University College and Middlesex School of Medicine, London

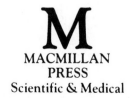
MACMILLAN
PRESS
Scientific & Medical

First published 1989

Published by
THE MACMILLAN PRESS LTD
Houndmills, Basingstoke, Hampshire RG21 2XS
and London
Companies and representatives
throughout the world

Typeset by
Ponting–Green Publishing Services, London

Printed in Hong Kong

ISBN 0–333–49109–2

CONTENTS

Section 3: The Larynx and Tracheobronchial Tree

Section 5: General and Related

FOREWORD

A great deal of work has gone into compiling these multiple-choice questions and answers. They are more interesting and entertaining than simply reading a text book, but are not, of course, an alternative.

At each stage in your study, take advantage of the questions section by section to see how much you have taken in. As the Americans say, 'frequent "mini exams" keep up the concentration'.

Not only students, but also all otolaryngologists will find this book worthwhile for occasional reading, to see how much they know or think they know. It will also be useful to those who have to set questions, whether multiple-choice or otherwise.

This book is something different and is certainly worthwhile. It does not take long to get used to the inevitable little tricks that multiple-choice questions present.

Richard A. Williams, MA, MB, BChir, FRCS, FRCS(E), DLO

Director,
Ferens Institute of Otolaryngology,
London
August 1988

PREFACE

Like them or loathe them, multiple-choice questions are firmly established in undergraduate and postgraduate medical education. Their importance can only increase as computers are used more and more to automate the assessment of students.

This book is designed primarily as a revision aid. It is particularly suitable for DLO and FRCS candidates throughout the world, but it could be used with profit by undergraduates. It can be used to discover gaps in knowledge and to reinforce what has been learned from standard textbooks. We have included short notes with the answers. These provide further information and try to explain why we favour a given response in cases where there may be disagreement.

There are 1590 questions here, arranged as 318 stems, each with 5 independent true/false statements. All major areas of otolaryngology are covered. The questions are ordered by subject in 5 sections: Ear; Nose and Sinusus; Larynx and Tracheobronchial Tree; Mouth; Pharynx and Oesophagus; and General and Related Subjects.

The subject matter is covered in the standard British ENT textbooks. We have made extensive use of Scott-Brown, both fourth and fifth editions, the ear, nose and throat volumes of Rob and Smith's *Operative Surgery*, Groves and Gray's *Synopsis of Otolaryngology*, Stell and Maran's *Head and Neck Surgery*, and Mawson and Ludman's *Diseases of the Ear.*

When compiling MCQs it is tempting to stick to factual or uncontroversial issues. This artificial restriction takes a lot of the interest out of the subject. We have included controversial aspects of clinical practice, as well as basic anatomy, physiology and pathology. We recognize that the reduction of complex issues to a series of true/false statements can never be perfect. No doubt some experienced colleagues will disagree with our answers. Perhaps they will take consolation from the fact that in real life the unfortunate candidate not only has to know what is right, but also to know what the examiner knows is right!

We are grateful to the Director and staff of the Ferens Institute of Otolaryngology, under whose auspices the book was produced. We also thank our colleagues and students at the Royal Ear Hospital, the Middlesex Hospital and Mount Vernon Hospital for their helpful suggestions. In particular we would like to thank Mr Richard Williams, Mr Graham Fraser, Mr Garry Glover and Mr Phillip Robinson for their careful reading of the questions. They have all pointed out ambiguities and inconsistencies which bedevil the MCQ compiler. Any faults which remain are the authors' responsibility. Finally, we would like to thank our wives, Georgina and Sylvia, for their continued support during the two-year gestation period of the book.

London, 1989   R.S.D.
                                                                                        J.W.F.

SECTION 1
THE EAR

1   In foetal development

A   There are 6 visceral arches and 5 visceral clefts.
B   The facial nerve supplies the second or hyoid arch.
C   The pharyngeal pouches are formed from the ectodermal
furrows.
D   The tuberculum impar, the lingual swellings and the
hypobranchial eminence form the tongue.
E   In the adult the sulcus terminalis in the tongue marks the site of
the thyroid rudiment.

2   Development of the foetal ear

A   The eustachian tube is formed from the ectoderm of the first
visceral cleft.
B   The auricle develops from the first visceral cleft as a series of 6
tubercles.
C   The stapes footplate is derived from ectoderm.
D   The inner ear is developed from ectoderm and has reached full
size by the 4th foetal month.
E   The stapes superstructure, styloid process and hyoid are
derived from the 1st visceral arch.

3   Development of the temporal bone

A   The tympanic ring and squama are ossified in cartilage.
B   The foramen of Huschke is a defect in the tympanic ring.
C   Ossification of the endosteal layer of the petromastoid may be
defective particularly in the vicinity of the fissula ante fenestram.
D   The facial nerve is well protected at birth by the mastoid
process.
E   In the infant the mastoid antrum lies below the tympanic cavity
and about 5 mm deep to the bony surface.

1

A   **F.**   There are 6 of each.

B   **T.**   Each visceral arch has its own nerve supply. The mandibular division of the trigeminal nerve supplies the mandibular arch (1st); the facial the hyoid arch (2nd); the glossopharyngeal (3rd); the vagus and accessory the remainder.

C   **F.**   They are formed from the endodermal furrows.

D   **T.**

E   **F.**   The site is the foramen caecum.

2

A   **F.**   Formed from the endoderm of the tubotympanic recess. The ectoderm of the first cleft forms the external auditory canal.

B   **T.**   These eventually fuse to form the definitive pinna.

C   **F.**   The stapes head, neck and crura are derived from mesoderm of the 2nd visceral arch and the footplate from the otic capsule. Hence otosclerosis, a disease of the otic capsule, primarily affects the footplate region.

D   **T.**

E   **F.**   Bone and cartilaginous derivatives are:
1st arch—malleus, incus, Meckel's cartilage
2nd arch—stapes, styloid process, stylohyoid ligament, greater part of hyoid body
3rd arch—hyoid inferior body and greater cornu
4th arch—thyroid and epiglottis
6th arch—arytenoids.

3

A   **F.**   Both are formed in membrane. The other 2 elements of the temporal bone are the styloid process (derived from cartilage of the 2nd arch) and the petromastoid (formed in cartilage).

B   **T.**   The incomplete tympanic ring grows asymmetrically leaving a deficiency in the external canal antero-inferiorly and so infection may spread between parotid and meatus.

C   **F.**   It is the thick middle layer of the petromastoid (enchondral layer) that may undergo defective ossification; particularly anterior to the oval window; a frequent site of otosclerotic foci.

D   **F.**   The mastoid is flat at birth and the stylomastoid foramen, through which the facial nerve emerges, is very superficial and is at risk from injury.

E   **F.**   It lies above and is only 2 mm deep. Hence the increased risk to the facial nerve and labyrinth during surgery.

4   Development of the mastoid process

A   The diploic type has large and numerous air cells containing marrow spaces.

B   Wittmaack suggested that disease processes, in particular infantile otitides, prevent normal mastoid pneumatization.

C   Diamant suggested that hypocellularity of the mastoid is merely a normal variant.

D   Both the Tumarkin and the mastoid plate distraction theories of mastoid pneumatization depend on satisfactory middle ear ventilation.

E   Only about 50% of mastoids are pneumatized.

5   Anatomy of the external ear

A   The auricular skin is loosely adherent to the underlying perichondrium of yellow elastic cartilage.

B   The external meatus has the temporomandibular joint as an anterior relation, the mastoid antrum posterosuperiorly and the middle cranial fossa superiorly.

C   The great auricular (C1 and C2), the vagus and the trigeminal nerves supply sensation.

D   The blood supply is from branches of the external carotid artery.

E   The lymphatics of the lobule drain to the external jugular lymph nodes.

6   In the adult

A   The external meatus is 25 mm long and the bony inner two thirds is directed medially and inferiorly.

B   The bony portion of the external meatus is lined by skin bearing glands and hairs.

C   The yellow elastic cartilage of the outer one third of the meatus is deficient superiorly.

D   Skin lining the bony meatus is closely adherent at the tympanomastoid and squamotympanic sutures.

E   The pain of meatal furunculosis is due to a mild osteitis.

4

A **F.**   In the diploic type the spaces are small with few marrow spaces.

B **T.**   Infection interfered with resorption of diploic tissue.

C **T.**

D **T.**   Tumarkin's theory—failure of aeration due to eustachian tube blockage. Distraction theory—the inner and outer plates of the mastoid are separated by muscle pull.

E **F.**   80% pneumatized: 20% diploic or sclerotic.

5

A **F.**   The skin is very closely adherent; hence the extreme pain of haematomata and the oedema of external otitis. This skin is loosely adherent in the region of the mastoid; a donor site for full thickness skin graft.

B **T.**   Condylar movements may be conducted to the cartilaginous meatus (Costen's syndrome).

C **F.**   The great auricular nerve is C2 and C3 (posterior surface pinna). Vagus (Arnold's nerve)—posterior meatus; Trigeminal (V3 auriculotemporal—anterior meatus). There is probably some supply to the concha from the facial nerve as evidenced by the site of vesicular eruption in herpes zoster oticus.

D **T.**   Auriculotemporal branch of superficial temporal artery and posterior auricular artery. Ultimately derived from the external carotid artery.

E **T**

6

A **T.**   The bony meatus is also narrower than the cartilaginous portion.

B **F.**   Only the skin lining the cartilaginous portion of the meatus contains these structures.

C **T.**   Between the lamina of the tragus and the crus of the helix. A defect exploited in the endaural incision.

D **T.**   This fact plus the thinness of the skin makes elevation of a tympanomeatal flap difficult in these areas.

E **F.**   The skin is closely adherent in the cartilaginous portion (hair follicle bearing area) leaving little room for expansion.

7   In the middle ear cleft
A   The lining is pseudo stratified columnar ciliated epithelium anteriorly but flat or cuboidal posteriorly.
B   The eustachian tube is 37 mm long, the upper two thirds consisting of bone and the lower one third of an incomplete ring of cartilage.
C   Active contraction of the tensor palati results in the nasopharyngeal orifice of the eustachian tube opening.
D   Due to the eustachian tube's shorter length, wider diameter and relatively more horizontal alignment in the infant the risk of ascending infection is increased.
E   The eustachian tube is actively closed by the action of the palatal muscles.

8   The anterior wall of the tympanic cavity
A   Contains the notch of Rivinus.
B   Is the site of the Glasserian fissure containing the tympanic artery and anterior ligament of the malleus.
C   The chorda tympani, supplying light touch and proprioception to the anterior two thirds of the tongue, leaves through the Canal of Hugier.
D   Contains the root of the processus cochleariformis round which passes the tensor tympani muscle.
E   Is perforated by caroticotympanic nerves and by the tympanic artery.

9   In the middle ear cleft
A   The tegmen tympani is a thin plate of petrous bone separating the cleft from the middle cranial fossa.
B   The facial recess lies deep to the vertical portion of the facial nerve canal.
C   The stapedius tendon is inserted into the head of the stapes.
D   The superficial landmark of the mastoid antrum is the suprameatal triangle.
E   The short process of the incus is attached by ligaments to the floor of the aditus.

7

A   **T.**   This difference is the basis for different pathological processes seen in chronic suppurative otitis media. Cuboidal region (atticoantral cholesteatoma): columnar region (tubotympanic disease).

B   **F.**   The upper one third is bony and the lower two thirds cartilage. The cartilaginous deficiency is bridged by fibrous connective tissue.

C   **T.**   Tensor palati takes origin from the lateral aspect of the cartilaginous part of the eustachian tube. The levator palati also acts to open the tube.

D   **T.**

E   **F.**   In the inactive or resting phase the tube is closed passively.

8

A   **F.**   This notch is the region where the pars flaccida is attached to the squamous portion of the temporal bone superiorly (the tympanic incisura).

B   **T.**   Also called the 'petrotympanic suture'. It connects the middle ear and temporomandibular and parotid regions. A potential route for the spread of infection.

C   **F.**   The chorda tympani does exit via the Canal of Hugier but carries only taste fibres from the anterior two thirds of the tongue.

D   **T.**   An important landmark for the first genu of the facial nerve.

E   **T.**   The nerves are derived from the sympathetic plexus on the internal carotid artery sheath.

9

A   **T.**   It is continuous with the tegmen antri.

B   **F.**   The sinus tympani lies deep to it and may form a site for hidden cholesteatoma. The facial recess lies lateral to the vertical facial canal but deep to the tympanic annulus.

C   **F.**   Inserted into the neck.

D   **T.**   Otherwise called MacEwen's triangle. The antrum is approximately l.5 cm deep to it in the adult.

E   **T.**   The short process serves as a landmark to the horizontal semicircular canal (medial to it) and the facial nerve (inferomedial).

10 Mucosal folds, compartments and ligaments of the middle ear cleft

 A   They may limit infection.
 B   The pouch of Prussak lies between the neck of the malleus and pars flaccida.
 C   The posterior ligament of the incus connects the short process of the incus to the fossa incudis.
 D   The lateral ligament of the malleus is attached to the margin of the tympanic notch of Rivinus.
 E   The pouches of Von Tröltsch lie between the malleolar folds and the handle of the malleus.

11 The middle ear cleft

 A   The tegmen tympani and antri separate the middle ear cleft from the posterior cranial fossa.
 B   The horizontal and vertical portions of the facial nerve always traverse in bony canals.
 C   The V and VI cranial nerves may be affected by spreading middle ear disease.
 D   The jugular bulb may be located in the mesotympanum.
 E   The sigmoid portion of the lateral sinus is posteromedial to the mastoid process.

12 Neurovascular supply of the middle ear cleft

 A   The hypotympanum is supplied by the inferior tympanic artery.
 B   The internal carotid artery supplies the anterior mesotympanum.
 C   The postauricular artery supplies the mastoid air cells.
 D   Sensation is derived from the glossopharyngeal nerve.
 E   Both the vagus and cochleovestibular nerves give a motor supply to middle ear muscles.

10
A **T.**
B **T.**
C **T.**
D **T.**
E **T.**   The anterior pouch between the anterior malleolar fold and the tympanic membrane anterior to the handle. The posterior pouch between the posterior malleolar fold and the tympanic membrane posterior to the handle.

11
A **F.**   Separates the cleft from the middle cranial fossa and hence the temporal lobe. Erosion of the tegmen by atticoantral cholesteatoma may lead to intracranial complications.
B **F.**   The bony covering may be thin or dehiscent. Hence a greater risk to the nerve during surgery and otitis media.
C **T.**   Gradenigo's syndrome. (Ipsilateral facial pain, lateral rectus palsy and otorrhoea.)
D **T.**   If the tympanic cavity floor is dehiscent. May be at risk during myringotomy.
E **T.**   Hence the occasional spread of disease of the middle cleft leading to lateral sinus thrombophlebitis and otitic hydrocephalus.

12
A **T.**   The artery is a branch of the ascending pharyngeal artery which is the second branch of the external carotid.
B **T.**   Via a branch called the ramus tympanici which pierces the anterior wall.
C **T.**   Via its stylomastoid branch.
D **T.**   Via Jacobson's branch to the tympanic plexus. Hence referred otalgia from lesions of posterior third of tongue.
E **F.**   Trigeminal nerve supplies tensor tympani muscle, and the facial nerve (nerve to stapedius) supplies the stapedius muscle.

13 In the labyrinth
A   The orifice of the vestibular aqueduct is located in the anterior part of the medial wall of the bony vestibule.
B   The most superior part of the superior semicircular canal is located beneath the arcuate eminence.
C   In the anatomical position the plane of the lateral semicircular canals is at an angle of 30 degrees to horizontal, tilting down posteriorly.
D   The osseous labyrinth contains endolymph and the membranous labyrinth perilymph.
E   The scala media is also known as the cochlear duct.

14 In the inner ear
A   The scala tympani, containing endolymph, communicates with the subarachnoid space via the cochlear aqueduct.
B   Cortilymph is similar to perilymph.
C   There are 3–4 rows of outer hair cells which are arranged in rows in a pattern of a W.
D   The inner hair cells are columnar in shape compared to the outer hair cells which are bulbous.
E   The stria vascularis is located on the outer aspect of the cochlear duct.

15 In the cochlear nerve
A   The type I fibres are probably efferent and type II probably afferent.
B   The dorsal root ganglion is represented by the spiral ganglion and the nerve by the central processes.
C   The first synapse is at the dorsal and ventral cochlear nuclei after which the majority of fibres ascend in the contralateral lateral lemniscus.
D   The primary auditory centres are located in the trapezoid body.
E   The olivocochlear fibres are type II fibres, originate from both olivary nuclei and terminate at the base of the cochlea.

16 In the vestibular labyrinth
A   The three semicircular ducts open into the utricle by six separate openings.
B   The utriculo-endolymphatic valve consists of flaps of mucosa permitting inflow and not outflow of endolymph.
C   The macula of the utricle lies in the horizontal plane and that of the saccule in a vertical plane.
D   The hair cells of the utricular macula project into a membrane containing otoliths.
E   Depolarization of a sensory cell occurs if the stereocilia are displaced away from the kinocilium.

13

A **F.** Located in the posterior wall and so lies on the posterior surface of the petrous bone. The aqueduct contains the endolymphatic duct and a small vein.

B **T.**

C **T.** Hence a patient is lain supine with the head tilted 30 degrees upwards to perform caloric tests. This position brings the lateral canals into a vertical plane which is most sensitive to a thermal gradient.

D **F.** The reverse is true. A perilymph leak may be produced by opening the bony labyrinth, e.g. at stapedectomy or rupture of the round window membrane.

E **T.** It is the portion of the membranous labyrinth containing endolymph.

14

A **F.** It contains perilymph. The intracranial communication is correct and may be route of pressure transmission from cranium to the inner ear leading to round window ruptures.

B **T.** It may be derived from the scala tympani via foramina in the osseous spiral lamina.

C **T.**

D **F.** The reverse is true.

E **T.**

15

A **F.** Type I fibres (23 000–40 000) are sparsely granulated and afferent. Type II fibres (500–600) are richly granulated, efferent and originate in the superior olivary nucleus.

B **T.**

C **T.**

D **F.** Located in the pons (medial geniculate body and inferior colliculus).

E **T.** One fifth are homolateral; four fifths are contralateral. These olivocochlear fibres may be responsible for fine tuning the cochlear and have been implicated in the production of cochlear echoes and tinnitus.

16

A **F.** There are only five openings as the posterior and superior canals have a common crus into the utricle.

B **F.** The valvular action is produced by the acute angle formed as the endolymphatic duct leaves the utricle.

C **T.** The macula is sensory epithelium and in the semicircular canals is represented by the crista of each ampulla.

D **T.** The hair cells are embedded in the statoconial membrane which contains calcite particles (statoconia).

E **F.** This causes hyperpolarization and a reduction in firing rate of vestibular nerve fibres.

17 The vestibular nerve
A   Scarpa's ganglion is located in the internal auditory canal.
B   There are anastamotic connections between the superior vestibular nerve and facial nerve.
C   The inferior vestibular nerve supplies the posterior canal and the saccule.
D   The vestibular nuclei send fibres to the medial longitudinal bundle (MLB) which are responsible for reflex postural muscle tone.
E   The blood supply is mainly from the internal auditory artery which is derived from the posterior inferior cerebellar artery.

18 Blood supply of the labyrinth
A   The internal auditory artery divides into an anterior vestibular and common cochlear branches.
B   The cochlear artery ultimately forms the stria vascularis.
C   The spiral modiolar artery has rich anastamoses with terminal branches of the vestibulocochlear artery.
D   The vestibulocochlear artery is a branch of the common cochlear.
E   The labyrinthine artery is the principal arterial supply of the inner ear.

19 Anatomy of the internal auditory canal
A   The fundus, at the lateral end, is a vertical plate of thin solid bone.
B   The transverse crest separates the inferior vestibular nerve from the cochlear nerve.
C   'Bill's' bar or the vertical crest was named after King William IV of England.
D   The vertical crest divides the upper compartment into an anterior portion for the facial nerve and a posterior portion for the superior vestibular nerve.
E   The foramen singulare in the lower compartment, transmits the nerve from the posterior semicircular canal.

17

A **T.** In a vestibular neurectomy the transection should be sited <u>proximal</u> to the ganglion otherwise there is a risk of regeneration of nerve fibres.

B **T.** Via the nerve of Oort.

C **T.** The posterior ampullary branch can be sectioned (singular neurectomy) for treatment of the severe protracted form of benign paroxysmal positional vertigo. It is approached through the middle ear.

D **F.** Vestibular fibres to the MLB influence the 3rd, 4th and 6th nerve nuclei and hence the extrinsic ocular muscles. The vestibulospinal tract is responsible for muscle tone.

E **F.** The internal auditory artery is a branch of the anterior inferior cerebellar but may arise directly from the basilar.

18

A **T.** The internal auditory is usually derived from the anterior inferior cerebellar artery but may arise directly from the basilar artery.

B **T.** The stria may be the site of both formation and absorption of endolymph and hence the source of electrical potentials in the inner ear.

C **F.** The spiral modiolar artery is an end artery and obstruction to its blood flow is a potential cause of sudden sensorineural deafness.

D **T.**

E **T.** Also called the internal auditory artery.

19

A **F.** The plate contains numerous perforations that transmit the fibres of vestibulocochlear and facial nerves.

B **F.** It divides the IAC into a small upper compartment (facial and superior vestibular nerves) from a larger lower compartment (cochlear and inferior vestibular nerves).

C **F.** Named after William House of the House Ear Institute, Los Angeles.

D **T.**

E **T.** This nerve is occasionally sectioned in persistent severe cases of benign paroxysmal positional vertigo (singular neurectomy).

20 Sensory nerve supply of the ear

A   The lesser occipital nerve (C1) supplies the upper medial surface of the pinna.
B   The 'Alderman's nerve' may be stimulated by instilling spirit or instruments into the external meatus.
C   The glossopharyngeal nerve supplies sensory fibres to the middle ear cleft.
D   The mandibular nerve supplies sensation to the lateral surface of the pinna and the anterior halves of the external meatus and tympanic membrane.
E   The seventh cranial nerve gives a sensory supply to the ear.

21 The following lesions may cause referred otalgia

A   Fibrositis of the upper portion of the sternomastoid muscle via the fibres of C2 and C3.
B   A high septal deviation causing pressure on the middle turbinate.
C   Parotid and submandibular calculi.
D   Acute sphenoidal and maxillary sinusitis.
E   An elongated styloid process.

22 The following neoplasms may present with otalgia

A   Nasopharyngeal carcinoma.
B   Tonsillar carcinoma.
C   Oesophageal carcinoma
D   Oropharyngeal carcinoma.
E   Chemodectoma of the larynx.

20

A **F.** The area supplied is correct but the lesser occipital is derived from C2. C1 has no sensory fibres. Referred otalgia via this nerve may occur in pathologies of the cervical vertebrae.

B **T.** Also called Arnold's nerve (auricular branch of the vagus). Instrumentation occasionally causes coughing paroxysms. The nerve supplies the posterior half of the external meatus and tympanic membrane. Instillation of spirit is said to enhance the appetite by reflex vagal stimulation and was carried out by Aldermen to increase their capacity for banqueting.

C **T.** Via the tympanic plexus derived from the tympanic branch of the glossopharyngeal nerve. Site of tympanic neurectomy for gustatory sweating occurring after parotid surgery.

D **T.** Via its auriculotemporal branch. Hence a cause of referred otalgia produced by petrous apex pathology (acoustic nerve tumours, primary cholesteatoma, etc), which irritates the trigeminal nerve.

E **T.** Based on the earache and conchal lesions produced by herpes zoster oticus (Ramsay Hunt syndrome).

21

A **T.**

B **T.** Via the trigeminal nerve. This pathology may also give rise to facial pain (Sluder's neuralgia).

C **T.** Via the trigeminal nerve.

D **T.** Via the trigeminal nerve.

E **T.** It stretches the glossopharyngeal nerve as it routes round the process. Causes stabbing pain in the side of the oropharynx and ear during mastication. The styloid process can usually be palpated in the tonsillar fossa and is readily visualized on plain X-rays.

22

A **T.** By ulceration and invasion of the mandibular division of the trigeminal as it emerges through the foramen ovale.

B **T.** Referred otalgia via the glossopharyngeal nerve.

C **T.** Rarely, via the vagus nerve. Particularly if the lesion has involved the recurrent laryngeal nerve coursing in the tracheo-oesophageal groove: pharyngeal neoplasia causes referred otalgia early in its evolution.

D **T.** Via the glossopharyngeal and vagus nerves.

E **T.** An unusual tumour but causes severe local pain and referred otalgia.

23 In the physical examination of the ear
A   The pars tensa is normally a blue-red colour.
B   Mobility of the ear drum can be assessed by Siegle's speculum.
C   The pars flaccida is also known clinically as the 'attic'.
D   The pars tensa is O.25 mm thick.
E   The lower end of the eustachian tube may be inspected directly using a rigid pharyngoscope passed through the mouth.

24 Radiological investigation of the petrous temporal bone
A   The fronto-occipital view allows a comparison of both mastoid processes and petrous bones.
B   Conventional tomography is excellent for viewing the facial canal and labyrinth.
C   Digital subtraction angiography (DSA) is more hazardous than direct puncture arteriography.
D   Gadolinium is an enhancing agent used in magnetic resonance imaging.
E   Computerized axial tomography results in similar radiation exposure levels as polytomography.

23

A **F.**   Normally light grey. It's commonly blue in cases of glue ear, haemotympanum, high jugular bulb and cholesterol granuloma.

B **T.**   Also with a pneumatic attachment to an electric auriscope. The Valsalva and Toynbee manoeuvres are also useful tests of mobility and eustachian tube function.

C **T.**   Although 'attic' is the most frequently used term for this region it is strictly that part of the middle ear cleft above the pars flaccida. Epitympanum and attic are synonyms.

D **F.**   Only 0.1 mm. The pars flaccida, not having a middle fibrous layer, is even thinner.

E **F.**   Can be viewed with a fibreoptic nasendoscope, rigid nasopharyngoscope, Yankauer postnasal space speculum or a St. Clair Thompson mirror.

24

A **T.**   Useful in cases of suspected apical petrositis and acoustic neuroma.

B **T.**   Tomography can be performed in several planes, e.g. axial, lateral (for visualization of the vestibular aqueduct), AP and PA. The disadvantage is the high radiation exposure to the orbit.

C **F.**   DSA is safer and provides information almost as detailed as traditional arteriography.

D **T.**   Enhances many types of neoplasia, including acoustic neuromata.

E **F.**   CAT scanning exposure is less. It is superior in revealing bone erosion and of course provides additional information regarding midline shift and visualization of the brain stem.

25 The following procedures are usually performed via a permeatal incision

- A   Exploration of the vertical portion of the facial nerve.
- B   Membranous labyrinthectomy for Menière's disease.
- C   Tympanic neurectomy.
- D   Cochlear implantation.
- E   Fenestration of the lateral semicircular canal.

26 In temporal bone surgery

- A   The suprameatal triangle is the surface landmark of the mastoid antrum.
- B   The endaural incision divides tragal cartilage at the incisura terminalis.
- C   All postaural incisions should be placed about 1 cm behind the postauricular sulcus and extend inferiorly to the tip of the mastoid process.
- D   Trautmann's triangle is part of the bony plate of the posterior cranial fossa.
- E   The bone over an infant's antrum is microscopically cribriform.

27 Principles of temporal bone surgery

- A   The radical mastoidectomy involves complete removal of the ossicles and tympanic membrane and lowering the posterior canal wall.
- B   In an attico antrostomy the only ossicle removed is the incus.
- C   Removal of bone in the antrum threshold angle allows access to the mesotympanum in a posterior tympanotomy.
- D   The solid angle is formed by bone in the angle between the three semicircular canals.
- E   In a Schwartze mastoidectomy the posterior canal wall is lowered.

25

A **F.** Only the horizontal portion of the facial is seen in this approach. A postauricular approach will allow exposure of the vertical portion.

B **T.** By turning the stapes with its footplate laterally, hooking out the saccule and instilling 100% alcohol to destroy any remaining neuroepithelium.

C **T.** In severe cases of gustatory sweating after parotid surgery (Frey's syndrome) which does not resolve spontaneously. Has also been advocated for reduction of drooling in cerebral palsy. As with other forms of autonomic surgery, the results are good initially but rarely last longer than 2 years.

D **F.** Entering the middle ear via a posterior tympanotomy is the usual approach.

E **F.** A virtually obsolete operation for otosclerosis since the introduction of stapedectomy. May be indicated in cases of persistent stapedial artery and inadequate access to the footplate due to abnormalities of the facial nerve.

26

A **T.** In an adult located I.5 cm deep to the landmark. Also called MacEwen's triangle.

B **F.** No cartilage is divided hence a reduced risk of perichondritis.

C **F.** In infants and young children the inferior extension should be very limited to avoid damage to the superficially placed facial nerve. The mastoid process does not appear until the second year of life.

D **T.** Bounded posteriorly by the sigmoid sinus, anteriorly by the bony labyrinth (posterior semicircular canal) and superiorly by the superior petrosal sinus.

E **T.** Hence an acute otitis media is actually a subperiosteal infection.

27

A **F.** The stapes footplate with or without the superstructure is preserved.

B **F.** Both the incus and malleus head are removed.

C **T.** The angle boundaries are: medially, the vertical portion of the facial nerve; laterally, the chorda tympani and superiorly, the fossa incudis. It is in effect a dissection of the facial recess.

D **T.** It is medial to the mastoid antrum.

E **F.** Wide exenteration of all mastoid air cells is performed but the canal wall is left intact. Also called cortical or conservative mastoidectomy.

28 The seventh cranial nerve
A   The intracranial segment can be exposed through a posterior fossa craniectomy.
B   The stylomastoid foramen can be visualized in the submentovertical view of the skull base.
C   The junction of the facial canal with the lateral semicircular canal is usually marked by a mucosal vein.
D   The anterior end of the digastric ridge is a useful landmark for the stylomastoid foramen.
E   The main trunk is usually divided and grafted during superficial parotidectomy.

29 Physical properties of sound
A   Frequency is subjectively perceived as pitch.
B   Intensity and loudness are related to sound energy.
C   The reference intensity pressure in audiometry is 0.024 dyne/cm^2 at 100 Hz.
D   Overtones are multiples of the fundamental note.
E   White noise is produced by many frequencies at different intensities.

30 Sound transmission in the middle ear
A   The intact tympanic membrane protects the round window and directs sound energy to the ossicular chain and oval window.
B   The ossicular leverage action ratio of the malleus and incus is about 1.3:1.
C   The mode of vibration of the stapes changes with high sound intensities.
D   The physiological ratio of tympanic membrane to oval window surface area is about 21:1.
E   The transformer ratio of the ossicular chain plus the tympanic membrane is about 18:1.

31 Middle ear acoustic impedance
A   An increase in the stiffness of the vibrating parts produces frequency-selective deafness.
B   The presence of fluid affects mainly the high frequencies.
C   Ossicular chain discontinuity with an intact tympanic membrane results in a reduced middle ear compliance.
D   Otosclerosis and adhesive otitis media increase the stiffness of the vibrating parts.
E   Tympanosclerosis increases the middle ear compliance.

28

A **T.**
B **T.**
C **T.**
D **T.**
E **F.**   The aim is to preserve the nerve intact.

29

A **T.**
B **T.**
C **F.**   It is 0.00024 dyne/cm^2 at 1000 Hz.
D **T.**   Subjectively perceived as quality or timbre. The
              fundamental note is the frequency of the lowest note.
E **F.**   It is a range of frequencies of similar intensities.

30

A **T.**   Sound energy is preferentially transmitted to the oval
              window. The eardrum acting as a baffle preventing
              sound reaching the round window.
B **T.**   The axis of rotation being a line joining the anterior
              process of the malleus and short process of the incus.
C **T.**   With low intensity sounds the axis is near the posterior
              margin of the footplate. At high intensity the axis runs
              longitudinally through the footplate. The latter affords
              greater protection of delicate inner ear structures.
D **F.**   The anatomical ratio is 21:1 but the tympanic
              membrane is fixed at its periphery. Only two thirds is
              available for physiological vibration. Therefore the
              physiological ratio is about 14:1.
E **T.**   This allows some degree of impedance matching
              between the external air and inner ear fluids.

31

A **T.**   Changes in stiffness mainly affect the lower
              frequencies.
B **F.**   Mainly the low frequencies due to increased stiffness
              (reduced compliance).
C **F.**   The compliance is increased.
D **T.**   Leading to a reduced compliance.
E **F.**   Reduces compliance by increasing the stiffness of the
              vibrating parts.

32 Abnormalities of middle ear function
A   Loss of the transformer mechanism alone produces a hearing loss of about 50 dB.
B   A round window baffle effect in modified radical mastoidectomy may allow a hearing threshold within 25 dB of normal.
C   A columellar effect is produced by conservation of only the ossicular chain lever ratio of the transformer mechanism.
D   No sound is perceived by air conduction if there is total loss of the middle ear mechanism.
E   A blast injury may increase middle ear compliance.

33 Middle ear muscles
A   Reflex contraction to sound stimulus is ipsilateral.
B   Contractions may be audible.
C   The stapedius and tensor tympani produce opposite effects on the drumhead.
D   Contraction attenuates the middle and high frequencies.
E   Contraction allows protection against acoustic trauma due to explosions.

34 Hearing by bone conduction
A   The skull vibrates.
B   The mandible may have a role.
C   Is used as a measure of cochlear function.
D   The compression theory applies to hearing sounds of higher frequencies.
E   Below 800 Hz the skull vibrates as a whole.

32

A **F.** Only 25–30 dB loss (round window protection maintained).

B **T.** Although the transformer mechanism is lost the preferential sound conduction to the oval windows is maintained. Hence only a 25 dB loss instead of the expected 40–60 dB loss.

C **F.** The ossicular chain lever ratio is lost and the areal ratio of the drumhead and oval window preserved.

D **F.** The basilar membrane moves due to yielding of inner ear contents.

E **T.** If ossicular disconnection has occurred.

33

A **F.** The reflex is consensual.

B **T.** Particularly of the tensor tympani: a cause of objective tinnitus.

C **T.** The tensor displaces it medially and the stapedius laterally.

D **F.** Attenuates the more damaging low frequencies allowing preferential transmission of the middle and high frequencies.

E **F.** The latency of the muscle reflexes means that they cannot contract in time to protect against high intensity noise of sudden onset.

34

A **T.** Effective stimuli include the subject's own voice, ambient sound pressures and direct contact with a vibrating object as in tuning fork tests.

B **T.** It produces vibrations due to inertia of the cartilaginous meatus, which are transmitted by the normal air conduction route to the inner ear. Other theories of bone conduction include the inertia of the ossicular chain and compression of labyrinthine fluids.

C **T.** Tuning fork tests and bone conduction audiometry.

D **T.** Both the fronto-occipital and biparietal diameters alter during higher frequency stimulation. This causes compressional activity in the labyrinth.

E **T.** Hearing therefore results from inertia of the ossicular chain allowing the stapes to oscillate in the oval window.

35 In the cochlea
A   The perilymph and cerebrospinal fluid are connected by the vestibular aqueduct.
B   The scala media has a resting electrical potential of + 80 mV.
C   Short travelling waves are produced by low pitched sound stimuli.
D   The cochlear microphonic is generated at the hair-cell tectorial membrane interface.
E   Summating potentials are predominantly produced by outer hair cell activity.

36 Theories of hearing
A   Helmholtz suggested a precise place of vibration of the basilar membrane for each frequency.
B   The 'telephone theory' suggested a simple 1:1 ratio of frequency of sound stimuli and firing of nerve action potentials.
C   Wever suggested that between 400 and 5000 Hz groups of nerve fibres fired in temporal sequence.
D   The volley theory states that frequencies above 5000 Hz are heard by the place principle.
E   Loudness appreciation may be increased by the action of outer hair cells.

37 Localization of sound stimulus
A   Interaural phase differences are important for low frequencies.
B   Complex sounds and transients are detected by differences in time of arrival at the ears.
C   The head produces a shadow effect on sound.
D   Monaural hearing is more efficient than binaural hearing.
E   Interaural intensity differences are important for frequencies above 1400 Hz.

38 In testing the hearing
A   The 1024 Hz tuning fork is best for general use.
B   Masking the good ear in severe unilateral sensorineural deafness is essential.
C   The Weber test always lateralizes to the better ear in sensorineural deafness.
D   The Gellé test is abnormal in conductive deafness.
E   In normal ears the Rinne test is usually neutral.

35

A **F.**   Connected by the cochlear aqueduct. Perilymph is probably a blood filtrate and has a different composition to CSF.

B **T.**

C **F.**   The short wave has its maximum displacement near the basal turn of the cochlea and is produced by high frequencies. Low frequencies nearer the apex.

D **T.**   It is absent if the hair cells are damaged, e.g. by aminoglycosides such as streptomycin.

E **F.**   The SP is produced by inner hair cell activity in response to high frequency sound stimuli.

36

A **T.**   The basilar membrane acting as a series of tuned resonators. Not feasible as the BM is highly damped.

B **T.**   Proposed by Rutherford. However, nerve latency periods allow this mechanism to operate only below 1000 Hz.

C **T.**   The ultimate signal presented to the auditory cortex being the actual frequency of the stimulus.

D **T.**   Hair cells in the basal turn only being stimulated.

E **T.**   Outer hair cells may effect a lowering of threshold of inner hair cells.

37

A **T.**   Particularly below 1400 Hz.

B **T.**

C **T.**   Particularly of high frequencies and thus produces interaural intensity differences.

D **F.**

E **T.**

38

A **F.**   The 512 Hz is most useful. Below 256 Hz the vibrations are felt rather than heard; above 1024 Hz they fade too rapidly.

B **T.**   Otherwise a false negative Rinne may be elicited. Hence the use of a Barany box. Masking is essential during audiometric threshold assessment.

C **F.**   May not in long-standing sensorineural deafness.

D **T.**   Alternating finger pressure on the ipsilateral tragus produces fluctuations of the sound of a tuning fork on the mastoid in cases of normal hearing and sensorineural deafness. There is no change in cases of conductive losses such as in ossicular discontinuity and fixation.

E **F.**   Is positive, AC better than BC.

39 In non-organic hearing loss

A Electrocochleography is essential to detect any thresholds.
B The stapedial reflex is seldom of value.
C Serial audiograms are usually inconsistent.
D The Chimani-Moos test is a modification of the Weber test.
E The Stenger test can be performed with either 2 tuning forks or an audiometer.

40 Audiological investigations

A Masking for air conduction is necessary if the hearing loss of the test ear exceeds 50 dB.
B A retrocochlear deafness gives a speech discrimination far better than expected from pure tone thresholds.
C Carhart's test is a measure of tone decay.
D Recruitment is uncommon in both cochlear and neural hearing losses but usual in conductive losses.
E Loudness reversal elicited in the Fowler test indicates neural deafness.

39

A **F.** Thresholds can be estimated without any electrical tests. The non-invasive brainstem evoked response (BSER) or cortical electrical response audiometry (CERA) are more widely used than ECochG.

B **F.** It is a useful objective test provided it is used in conjunction with other audiological investigations.

C **T.** Also a shadow audiogram of an unmasked 'good' ear is rarely produced. In a genuine case, the shadow audiogram would be expected with stimuli in excess of 50 dB applied to the deaf ear.

D **T.** The malingerer hears the tuning fork in the good ear and may say he hears nothing when the same ear is occluded.

E **T.** The principle is that two tones of equal frequency cannot be heard if one is louder than the other.

40

A **T.** At this level sounds may be conducted to the non-test ear by skull vibrations. Masking is necessary in all bone conduction measurements and consists of narrow-band filtered white noise centered on the test frequency.

B **F.** Classically the speech discrimination score is very poor. Cochlear deafness produces the 'roll over' effect where the speech score deteriorates with increasing intensity levels.

C **T.** A decay of more than 30 dB may be seen in neural deafness, particularly significant if elicited at 500 Hz and/or 1000 Hz.

D **F.** Not seen in conductive deafness: very common in cochlear lesions and seen in about 10% of retrocochlear lesions (acoustic neuromata particularly).

E **T.** Fowler's test is the 'Alternate binaural loudness balance test'.

41 Impedance audiometry
A   Ossicular discontinuity is best illustrated using a 660 Hz probe tone.
B   The stapedial reflex is usually lost before the compliance is reduced in cases of otosclerosis.
C   A patulous eustachian tube produces a flat tympanogram.
D   Stapedius reflex decay at 4000 Hz indicates a retrocochlear disorder.
E   An impedance value of over 2 ml on a tympanogram may indicate the presence of a pin-hole perforation of the drumhead.

42 Electric response audiometry
A   A large summating potential on electrocochleography is a reflection of hair cell damage.
B   Over 90% of acoustic neuromata will reveal an interaural latency difference of the fifth wave of greater than 0.4 ms with brain stem electrical responses.
C   The postauricular myogenic responses give a very accurate measure of hearing thresholds in young children.
D   Electrocochleography can produce responses to stimuli of 250 Hz or less.
E   General anaesthesia affects the responses obtained during brainstem electrical stimulation.

41

A **T.** The tympanogram may be double peaked. With a 220 Hz probe tone the compliance is shown to be increased.

B **T.** If the maximum compliance is less than 0.3 ml a type 3 or 4 footplate is said to be likely.

C **F.** There are fluctuations of compliance in phase with respiratory movements.

D **F.** A decay of more than half the amplitude in 5 s at 500 Hz or 1000 Hz is suggestive of a retrocochlear lesion.

E **T.** The same measurement may be obtained with a patent grommet but only if the eustachian tube is blocked. This figure is the compliance value of the whole middle ear cleft.

42

A **T.** The SP may swamp the usual diphasic action potential and the cochlear microphonic may also be abnormal.

B **T.** A correction factor is necessary if there is a marked hearing deficit. There is a small false positive rate. However, surgery would only be contemplated if a tumour is demonstrated radiologically.

C **F.** A positive response merely indicates the integrity of the neural pathway.

D **F.** Stimuli below 1000 Hz produce poor responses and are unreliable.

E **F.** Not affected by sedatives or general anaesthesia. Hence its value in measuring thresholds in the young and uncooperative patient or cases of suspected non-organic hearing loss.

43 Assessment of hearing thresholds in young children

 A   Distraction tests can be performed below 6 months of age.
 B   Conditioned techniques can be useful from 2 to 4 years.
 C   Reliable pure tone audiometry can usually be performed at a mental age of 4 years.
 D   A hearing aid can be used to assess hearing ability.
 E   Blinking, frowning and stilling are responses to sound of a normal 3 month child.

44 Electronic hearing aids

 A   In NHS aids the letter 'L' denotes a high frequency emphasis with a low frequency cut-off.
 B   A low frequency cut may be very useful in severe high frequency losses.
 C   Vented earmoulds are useful for 'ski slope' type audiograms.
 D   Peak clipping in sensorineural hearing loss with a reduced dynamic range may lead to distortion.
 E   The switch marked 'T' is for use in the presence of an inductive loop system.

43

A **F.** Distraction tests are useful between 6 and 24 months. The stimuli employed are a high frequency rattle (8000 Hz): low hum (500 Hz): a whispered 'S' (2–4000 Hz). An electronic device producing warble tones is also an effective stimulus. The test requires two people, a tester and a distractor who engages the child's attention. Head turning occurs toward the sound stimulus which is presented out of sight of the child at known intensities. A reasonably accurate audiogram can be constructed in most cases.

B **T.** These involve 'Go' games or specific responses to sound stimuli such as pitch pipes.

C **T.** The mental and not chronological age is important. At a mental age of 4 years children should be able to give reliable responses to PTA.

D **T.** Particularly if no response is obtained with drums and other loud noises.

E **T.**

44

A **F.** 'L' denotes low frequency emphasis (high frequency cut) 'H' denotes high frequency emphasis (low frequency cut) 'N' denotes normal (widest frequency response).

B **T.** Especially where the low frequency energy causes loudness discomfort i.e. recruitment. This is particularly seen in presbyacusis.

C **T.** This earmould construction allows emphasis of high frequency sounds. May give relief to the 'blocked up' feeling of a closed mould. Acoustic feedback is a problem with vented moulds.

D **T.** AGC (Automatic Gain Control) may prevent loudness discomfort levels being reached but there is a delay of onset of about 50 ms. However, distortion is not usually a problem with AGC.

E **T.** Loop systems are frequently installed in educational establishments, theatres and television sets.

45 Vestibular labyrinthine physiology
A   The utricular macula responds to angular acceleration.
B   Bithermal caloric responses are abolished in conditions of zero gravity.
C   Ampullofugal displacement of the cupula of the superior semicircular canal increases vestibular nerve activity.
D   The saccular maculae lie in a horizontal plane.
E   Steady rotation is detected by the semicircular canals.

46 Vestibular function tests
A   In the bithermal caloric test the ears are irrigated for 40 s with water, 5° Celsius above and below normal body temperature.
B   Rotation to the left indicates a labyrinthine disorder on the ipsilateral side during Unterberger's test.
C   In gait tests the subject tends to deviate to the affected side.
D   An abnormal optokinetic nystagmus usually indicates a central vestibular problem.
E   Doll's head eye movements are lost with lesions of the basal ganglia.

47 Bithermal caloric test
A   The fixation index compares the duration of nystagmus with and without optic fixation.
B   Decreased responses always indicate pathology.
C   Enhanced responses may be seen in cerebellar lesions.
D   Frenzel's glasses abolish optic fixation.
E   Water is introduced into the ear using a Dundas Grant coiled copper tube.

45

A **F.**   The utricular macula lies in the horizontal plane and therefore responds to tilt and linear acceleration.

B **T.**   The thermally induced changes in the specific gravity of the endolymph are no longer effective stimuli.

C **T.**   Ampullopetal displacement in the lateral semicircular canal.

D **F.**   Lie in a vertical plane. May be concerned with the detection of low frequency vibration.

E **F.**   Only increases or decreases are detected. Constant rotational rates do not stimulate the semicircular canals.

46

A **F.**   The irrigation time is correct. Water temperature is 7 ° Celsius above and below normal body temperature (44° and 30°).

B **T.**

C **T.**   Sensitivity of the tests is improved by closing the eyes or walking across a mattress. These manoeuvres abolish proprioceptive input.

D **T.**   Cortical or subcortical lesions.

E **F.**   Loss indicates severe brainstem pathology.

47

A **T.**

B **F.**   Decreased or absent responses may be due to habituation, e.g. ballet dancers and acrobats.

C **T.**   Both in amplitude and/or in duration. Usually with an ipsilateral directional preponderance.

D **F.**   Only reduce fixation. For complete abolition either use Frenzel's glasses with an infrared viewer or ENG in darkness.

E **F.**   The Dundas Grant tube is employed in a cold air caloric test for cases with eardrum perforations and mastoid cavities.

48 Electronystagmography
A   Measures changes in the corneo-vestibular electrical potentials.
B   May show multiple square waves in cerebellar disorders.
C   In a normal subject shows smooth sinusoidal waves on pendulum eye-tracking.
D   Is unable to give a measure of the amplitude of nystagmus.
E   Can only record nystagmus that is visible to the naked eye.

49 Congenital abnormalities of the external ear
A   Are due to a developmental failure of the 1st and 2nd elements of the branchial system.
B   Include collaural fistulae which may be closely related to the glossopharyngeal nerve.
C   May be associated with accessory auricles and microtia.
D   May produce Darwin's tubercle.
E   Are not associated with middle ear malformations.

50 Haematoma Auris
A   Has vegetable connotations.
B   Is due to extravasation of blood in the subcutaneous tissue plane.
C   Is treated initially by aspiration with a wide bore needle.
D   Should be treated by warming the pinna.
E   Can cause loss of cartilage support of the auricle.

48

A	**F.**	Detects changes in the corneo-retinal electrical field.
B	**T.**	It may also reveal ocular dysmetria. On command for lateral gaze the eyes overshoot the target.
C	**T.**	Ataxic eye tracking movements are highly suggestive of brainstem lesions.
D	**F.**	The ENG tracing should be calibrated before any test. It reveals both duration and amplitude of eye movements.
E	**F.**	Its advantage is that it may reveal visually undetectable nystagmus.

49

A	**T.**	
B	**F.**	Related to the facial nerve. Congenital aural fistulae are lined with squamous epithelium, usually opening near the ascending crus of the helix.
C	**T.**	Several first arch anomalies may be found in association with accessory auricles. The latter may be located anywhere from tragus to angle of mouth.
D	**T.**	A small elevation on the postero-superior part of the helix. An inherited condition that represents the tip of the mammalian ear.
E	**F.**	The 1st arch contributes to the malleus and incus and the 2nd arch to the stapes. Hence middle ear anomalies are quite common.

50

A	**T.**	Failure to treat the blood clot results in fibrosis with a deformity called 'a cauliflower ear'. A hazard of dedicated rugby forwards.
B	**F.**	The haemorrhage is between cartilage and perichondrium.
C	**T.**	But only if the haematoma is of recent onset. Otherwise a formal helical incision and suction is required.
D	**F.**	This treatment is for frost-bite of the auricle in its early stages and before gangrene has supervened.
E	**T.**	Due to devitalization of the cartilage or if a perichondritis supervenes as a result of surgical intervention or the haematoma becoming infected.

51 In otitis externa
A   Furunculosis may be misdiagnosed as acute mastoiditis.
B   Failure to resolve can be due to employing an inappropriate topical antibiotic preparation without aural toilet.
C   The mainstay of treating an acute infection is meatal toilet.
D   The conidiophores of an aspergillus niger fungal infection are easily identified on otoscopy.
E   When caused by dandruff selenium sulphide based shampoos are beneficial.

52 In malignant otitis externa
A   There is a spreading osteomyelitis of the temporal bone caused by *Haemophilus influenzae*.
B   The parotid gland is involved by direct extension of disease.
C   A purulent discharge coming through a tympanic perforation is commonly seen.
D   A urinalysis is indicated.
E   A Gradenigo syndrome may result.

53 Viral infections of the external ear
A   May be associated with cranial nerve palsies and encephalitis.
B   Otitis externa haemorrhagica may be associated with influenzal epidemics.
C   Otalgia and oropharyngeal discomfort may precede the rash in herpes zoster.
D   Acyclovir eradicates herpes infections.
E   Bullous myringitis is characterized by moderate pain.

51

A   **T.**   Particularly as the former may produce marked meatal swelling and postauricular oedema and tenderness. Furunculosis may be distinguished by eliciting pain on tragal pressure, enlargement of lymph nodes, postauricular tenderness (rather than over MacEwan's triangle) and clear mastoid air cells on X-ray.

B   **T.**   Can also be due to underlying chronic suppurative otitis media, fungal superinfection or sensitivity to the antibiotic preparation.

C   **T.**   Particularly of debris in the anterior meatal recess.

D   **T.**   As black specks. After meatal toilet 1% clo-trimazole or amphotericin cream can be applied.

E   **T.**   The external meatus being involved in essentially a scalp condition (Seborrhoeic otitis externa).

52

A   **F.**   The causative agent is usually *Pseudomonas aeruginosa*, although Bacteroides species have also been implicated.

B   **T.**   Extension occurs via the fissures of Santorini, which are natural clefts in the cartilaginous meatus.

C   **F.**   The eardrum is usually intact. The discharge arises from infection and granulations in the external meatus.

D   **T.**   Over 90% of patients are diabetics. Malnutrition, immunosuppression and extremes of age are other important aetiological factors.

E   **T.**   From involvement of the V and VI cranial nerves at the petrous apex. However the VII is the most commonly affected and is a bad prognostic sign. IX, X, XI and XII may be affected.

53

A   **T.**   Particularly with herpes zoster and may involve both the VII and XII nerves.

B   **T.**

C   **T.**   Usually by several days. The oropharyngeal symptoms are due to vesicles in the buccal mucosa and hard palate.

D   **F.**   Not effective against herpes virus harbouring in dorsal root ganglia. Systemic and topical preparations only shorten the period of symptoms.

E   **F.**   The pain is usually excruciating but settles quite rapidly.

54 Neoplastic disease of the external ear
A   Exostoses are the commonest benign tumours of the cartilage.
B   Ceruminomas are easily cured by simple excision.
C   Squamous carcinoma may be associated with xeroderma pigmentosa.
D   Basal cell carcinomas are usually seen in the external meatus.
E   An osteoma is composed of ivory bone.

55 In the external auditory meatus
A   Ceruminous and pilosebaceous glands are located in the cartilaginous meatus.
B   Keratosis obturans may be associated with bronchiectasis and sinusitis.
C   Chronic otitis externa may produce a fibrous stenosis.
D   Vegetable foreign bodies should be syringed with saline.
E   Live insects may be killed with insecticide spray.

56 Congenital anomalies of the middle ear cleft
A   Due to their common origin the outer, middle and inner ear elements are all effected.
B   Congenital conductive deafness with a normal meatus and eardrum is easily corrected surgically.
C   The Treacher–Collins syndrome is an expression of ear anomalies associated with other developmental defects of the 1st and 2nd branchial arches.
D   High definition CT scan is essential prior to any surgical intervention.
E   Wildervanck's syndrome is a conductive deafness associated with preauricular sinuses and appendages and auricular malformations.

54

A **F.** Origin is the bony canal. The sessile variety are related to cold water as seen in keen swimmers.

B **F.** Wide excision is required due to the frequency of local recurrence. May progress to adenocarcinoma.

C **T.** An inherited defect of an enzyme involved in repairing defective DNA.

D **F.** Most common on the auricle.

E **F.** Consists of cancellous or spongy bone. They are usually solitary and pedunculated. Exostoses are of ivory bone, multiple and sessile.

55

A **T.** As are hair follicles.

B **T.** Occurs in the younger age group. Appears as a cholesteatomatous mass in the deep meatus. Possibly due to reflex vagal stimulation of apocrine glands in the ear.

C **T.**

D **F.** Saline will cause them to swell. Employ surgical spirit or refer for microscopic suction clearance.

E **T.** Use only a short burst otherwise a caloric effect may be produced.

56

A **F.** The outer and middle ears are derived from elements of the 1st and 2nd branchial arches. The inner ear from the primordial otocyst. Anomalies may occur independently in the 2 groups.

B **F.** Usually the stapes and oval window are affected. The cochlea appears more fragile in these cases and so surgery is hazardous. If deafness has been present since early childhood it is often misdiagnosed as otosclerosis.

C **T.** Also called 'Mandibulofacial Dystosis' (Franceschetti–Zwahlen). Facial defects include hypoplastic malar bones, maxillae and mandible.

D **T.** Particularly to visualize the ossicles and the inner ear. Polytomography is also useful.

E **T.**

57 Surgery of congenital ear anomalies
A   The stapedius tendon is absent in 1% of cases.
B   The facial nerve takes an abnormal course in about 30% of cases and the fallopian canal is dehiscent in 6%.
C   A persistent stapedial artery, if present, usually crosses the stapes footplate posteriorly.
D   The malleus is the most commonly malformed ossicle.
E   An identifiable tragus is usually associated with a partially formed external meatus.

58 Surgical correction of congenital atresia of the external auditory meatus
A   Cases of unilateral atresia do not require investigation.
B   Exploration in bilateral cases can be deferred until about 4 years of age.
C   Plastic reconstruction of the auricle is relatively easy.
D   Restenosis of a reconstructed external canal is a frequent problem.
E   External ear remnants are good indicators of the location of the middle ear.

59 Traumatic perforation of the tympanic membrane
A   Blast rupture affects the pars flaccida.
B   Tinnitus and vertigo are permanent symptoms.
C   Blood clot should be syringed out immediately.
D   Myringoplasty should be performed as early as possible and always within the first 3 weeks.
E   Severe pain, requiring analgesia, continues for several days.

60 In basal skull fractures involving the petrous temporal bone
A   Longitudinal fractures are usually caused by blows to the occipital or frontal regions.
B   Transverse fractures commonly cause facial paralysis.
C   Haemotympanum may present as a blue or black eardrum.
D   Ecchymosis over the mastoid area may be present.
E   Sensorineural deafness is irreversible.

57

A	**T.**	Its absence has no consequence on sound transmission.
B	**T.**	A foreshortened trunk may rise superficial to the posterior annulus; if inferiorly displaced it runs across the promontory and rarely the main trunk may be bifid.
C	**F.**	Usually anteriorly.
D	**T.**	Frequently fused with the incus.
E	**T.**	Hence a greater chance of surgical success.

58

A	**F.**	It is imperative to check that hearing in the unaffected ear is normal. If it is not, rehabilitation must be instituted as soon as possible.
B	**T.**	Some advocate a bone conducting aid till age 4–5 years followed by surgical correction. Others argue that early correction as young as 2 years will allow better aiding and greater benefit for the acquisition of speech.
C	**F.**	May require several staged operations. The recently available Swedish prosthesis with titanium bone screws is superior to any result of plastic surgery.
D	**T.**	It may be associated with chronic infection. No single technique entirely prevents this complication.
E	**F.**	Not to be relied upon.

59

A	**F.**	Always the pars tensa.
B	**F.**	Usually transient.
C	**F.**	Never syringe.
D	**F.**	Many perforations will heal spontaneously. A minimum of 6 weeks should be allowed before intervening surgically.
E	**F.**	Pain is severe at the time of rupture but settles very rapidly thereafter. Persistent pain implies secondary infection.

60

A	**F.**	Usually temporal or parietal blows.
B	**T.**	The fracture line involves the labyrinth and internal auditory canal. Immediate and complete paralysis has a poor prognosis for recovery and may be an indication for urgent exploration via a middle cranial fossa approach.
C	**T.**	
D	**T.**	Due to bleeding into mastoid air cells (Battle's sign).
E	**T.**	Usually seen in cases of transverse fractures.

61 Otitic barotrauma
   A   Occurs in flying during descent rather than ascent.
   B   Is due to locking of the eustachian tube at a critical pressure
        difference of about 80 mm Hg.
   C   Commonly leads to hearing loss and autophony.
   D   Is more likely to occur in cases of mechanical obstruction in the
        nose.
   E   Resistant cases may require grommet insertion.

62 Acute suppurative otitis media
   A   The degree of mastoid pneumatization influences the clinical
        picture.
   B   Nasopharyngeal tumours are a very common aetiological factor.
   C   A subperiosteal abscess indicates infective spread beyond the
        bony cortex.
   D   Tenderness over the mastoid antrum is an important sign
        elicited by pressure applied in the postauricular sulcus.
   E   Antibiotics are mandatory.

61

A **T.**   When environmental pressure increases relative to middle ear pressure. Similar damage can occur in deep sea diving (during descent) and compression during hyperbaric radiotherapy.

B **T.**   At this pressure level the active muscular contraction is not able to open the eustachian tube.

C **T.**

D **T.**   Such as polyps, acute rhinitis, allergic rhinitis or simply a deviated septum.

E **T.**   Preventive measures include correction of nasal pathology; use of nasal vasoconstrictors, the Valsalva manoeuvre and chewing sweets prior to and during descents.

62

A **T.**   In high degrees of pneumatization a severe clinical course ensues due to the large mucosal surface area involved in the inflammation.

B **F.**   Although can occur in neoplasia of this site; acute rhinitis remains the most common precursor. Any process with the propensity for causing eustachian salpingitis can be implicated (sinusitis, nasopharyngitis).

C **T.**   Will occur more rapidly in a child due to the thinness of the bony cortex.

D **F.**   Elicited by palpation of MacEwen's triangle through the concha.

E **T.**   Should be appropriate to the infective organism and continued long enough to ensure complete resolution. Myringotomy is only rarely required. Nasal vasoconstrictors help reduce tubal congestion but have not been shown to influence outcome in controlled trials.

63 Acute petrositis
A   May form a parapharyngeal abscess.
B   Is a cause of Gradenigo's syndrome.
C   Frequently requires simple mastoidectomy.
D   Is of insidious onset and rarely causes pain or fever.
E   Can only occur in the 30% of petrous temporal bones which
     have air cells extending to the apex.

**64 Complications of acute inflammation of the middle ear cleft
     include**
A   Activation of quiescent cholesteatoma.
B   Destruction of middle ear ossicles.
C   Persistent eardrum perforations.
D   Acute mastoiditis.
E   Facial paralysis.

**65 Factors in the development and behaviour of chronic otitis
     media include**
A   Bone reaction including erosion and necrosis.
B   Disorder of middle ear ventilation.
C   Secondary bacterial infection
D   Reactions of the mucoperiosteal lining.
E   Infiltration by keratinizing stratified squamous epithelium.

63
A **T.** If the infection coalesces to form a petrous apex abscess which can tract caudally along the internal carotid artery.
B **T.** A triad of otorrhoea (continuing mastoid infection); diplopia, (VI cranial nerve involvement) and facial pain (irritation of the V cranial nerve).
C **F.** Usually resolves with aggressive antibiotic therapy. If surgery is performed all fistulous tracts must be followed to the petrous apex to provide adequate surgical drainage.
D **F.** Nearly always occurs in association with either acute otitis media or mastoiditis.
E **T.**

64
A **T.**
B **T.** But commoner in chronic infection.
C **T.**
D **T.** Bony necrosis of the bony septa of the mastoid air cell system which coalesce.
E **T.** Occurs in cases of dehiscent facial nerve canals. Invariably recovers as the acute infection is controlled either with antibiotic therapy or surgery (myringotomy, cortical mastoidectomy, etc.).

65
A **T.** In attico-antral chronic suppurative otitis media (CSOM).
B **T.** Particularly in non-suppurative otitis media (secretory otitis media).
C **T.** In both tubotympanic and attico-antral CSOM.
D **T.** Especially in tubotympanic CSOM where there is an increase in the columnar secreting (goblet) cells.
E **T.** In attico-antral (cholesteatomatous) CSOM.

66 Tubotympanic chronic suppurative otitis media (CSOM)
A   A non-marginal perforation of the pars tensa is usually present.
B   Middle ear polyps should be removed by the naked eye with a snare.
C   Cholesterol granulomata may occur.
D   Copious mucoid discharge is produced.
E   Adenoidectomy may be indicated.

67 Pathogenesis of acquired cholesteatoma
A   Congenital epidermoid rests may break through the outer attic wall.
B   Squamous epithelium from the external meatus can migrate through a marginal perforation.
C   Tumarkin's theory postulates an intratympanic negative middle ear pressure with collapse of the ear drum.
D   Prolonged infection of the middle ear cleft may lead to squamous metaplasia.
E   Bone erosion is mainly due to a pressure effect.

68 In attico-antral CSOM
A   Deafness is always marked if ossicular damage has occurred.
B   Copious malodorous otorrhoea is common.
C   Otalgia is commonly a presenting symptom.
D   A central perforation is invariable.
E   Vertigo is due to blockage of the eustachian tube.

66

A **T.** The hearing loss being greater if posteriorly placed
(round window unprotected) rather than anteriorly.

B **F.** An otomicroscope and forceps should be used. With a
snare there is increased risk of damage to the
ossicular chain. Without adequate visualization
attachment to the oval or round window or an
abnormal position of the facial nerve may not be noted.

C **T.** Consisting of cholesterol crystals, haemosiderin and
other blood pigments. One cause of a blue eardrum.

D **T.** Particularly profuse during upper respiratory tract
infections.

E **T.** To remove a physical or infective cause of tubal
occlusion.

67

A **T.** Although a possibility it is considered to be extremely
rare. The rests may be activated by an infective
episode.

B **T.** Immigration theory.

C **T.** Invagination of the pars flaccida with accumulation of
keratin which enters the attico-antral area after
secondary bacterial infection activates it.

D **T.**

E **F.** Enzymatic factors, and putrefying chronic infection are
the major causes.

68

A **F.** There may be a huge conductive loss but occasionally
the disease may bridge an ossicular gap—'silent
cholesteatoma'.

B **F.** Usually scanty. The offensive odour is due to the
osteitis with secondary infection.

C **F.** Hearing loss and otorrhoea are the usual symptoms.
Earache suggests a complication.

D **F.** The perforation is usually marginal but disease can
occur behind an intact eardrum.

E **F.** Indicates perilabyrinthitis and potential spread to the
inner ear; usually by fistularization of the lateral
semicircular canal and rarely the promontory.

69 Management of chronic suppurative otitis media with cholesteatoma

A   Intact canal wall mastoidectomy gives excellent access to the sinus tympani.

B   A posterior tympanotomy provides access to the mesotympanum and hypotympanum by dissection of the facial recess.

C   Combined approach tympanoplasty is the operation of choice where follow-up cannot be guaranteed.

D   A type III tympanoplasty may leave a residual hearing loss of about 25 dB.

E   No ossicles are sacrificed in a modified radical mastoidectomy.

70 Management of cholesteatoma in children is difficult because

A   Aural toilet is uncomfortable.

B   Primary epithelialization of mastoid cavities is usual.

C   There is a high frequency of nasopharyngeal infection.

D   Excessive fibrosis causes narrowing of the meatoplasty.

E   There is a high incidence of recurrence with combined approach tympanoplasty.

71 In an open mastoid cavity

A   Healing takes place by secondary intention.

B   Continuing otorrhoea may be due to an open eustachian tube.

C   Obliteration with bone pate is usually successful even in the presence of otorrhoea.

D   Complete eradication of cholesteatoma is not necessary if a pedicled muscle flap is used to obliterate the cavity.

E   Only about 40% heal satisfactorily.

72 Acute mastoiditis

A   There is a peak incidence around 11 years of age.

B   Citelli's abscess occurs in the sternomastoid muscle.

C   Sagging of the posterosuperior meatal wall is an important diagnostic sign.

D   Parenteral penicillin is the antibiotic of choice.

E   Schwartze operation may be required.

69

A **F.**   In this approach there is a high risk of leaving cholesteatoma in this site.

B **T.**

C **F.**   There is a very high recurrence rate. Most will require a 'second look' operation and ultimately may need an open procedure.

D **T.**

E **F.**   The incus and malleus head are removed.

70

A **T.**

B **F.**   Children produce excessive fibrogranular tissue, leading to chronically discharging cavities.

C **T.**   Especially up to age 11. Particular culprits are tonsils, adenoids and maxillary sinuses.

D **T.**   Due to an exuberant healing process.

E **T.**   The risk of recurrent cholesteatoma is so high with closed techniques that exteriorization despite the drawbacks above is preferred by many surgeons.

71

A **T.**   The raw bone surface is covered initially by vascular granulation tissue. Surface epithelium then grows in from the marginal meatal skin.

B **T.**   It may need to be sealed.

C **F.**   All active infection should be eradicated pre-operatively.

D **F.**   Essential to eradicate all disease.

E **F.**   Nearer 70% in experienced hands.

72

A **F.**   Like acute suppurative otitis media peak incidence is at about 6 years.

B **F.**   Extension of disease at the tip of the mastoid gives an abscess in the sternomastoid (Von Bezold's): if through the medial surface an abscess in the digastric triangle (Citelli's).

C **T.**   Frequently associated with a perforation and pus from the middle ear.

D **T.**   The infective organism is usually a beta haemolytic streptococcus. Watch out for the insidious type III pneumococcus.

E **T.**   Eponym for cortical or simple mastoidectomy performed to exenterate all mastoid air cells.

73 Intracranial extension of suppurative otitis media
A   Can occur by bone erosion by cholesteatoma.
B   May be through the petrosquamous suture line.
C   Via the labyrinth may extend along the aqueduct of the cochlea.
D   Through the mastoid emissary vein is possible.
E   Along a dehiscent facial canal is rare.

74 Complications of suppurative otitis media
A   Include retropharyngeal abscess.
B   Rarely involve the middle cranial fossa because of the resistance of the tegmen antri and tympani.
C   May give a positive Tobey–Ayer test.
D   Are more likely to give rise to otogenic intracranial hypertension with the left ear.
E   Include Luc's abscess.

75 Secretory otitis media (SOM)
A   Is most prevalent in the second decade.
B   In the infant is commonly due to an abnormal eustachian tube.
C   Is more likely in the presence of large infected adenoids.
D   Infection is an aetiological factor.
E   May be consequent upon inadequate antibiotic therapy for acute otitis media.

73

A   **T.**

B   If non-united. Less frequently through the squamomastoid or occipitomastoid sutures.

C   **T.**   Once in the labyrinth there are also preformed pathways along the internal auditory canal and the vestibular aqueduct.

D   **T.**   Also via vascular foraminae in MacEwan's triangle.

E   **T.**   But certainly possible.

74

A   **T.**   Or a parapharyngeal abscess as pus can track along peritubal cells.

B   **F.**   Both are frequent sites of extension of disease.

C   **T.**   In cases of occluding thrombus in the lateral venous sinus no rise in CSF on manometry is noted on ipsilateral internal jugular vein compression. It is a late sign.

D   **F.**   The superior sagittal sinus more frequently drains into the right lateral sinus. Retrograde thrombophlebitis blocking the arachnoid villi in the former sinus is the pathophysiological basis of otitic hydrocephalus.

E   **T.**   Extension of infection under the periosteum of the roof of the bony canal to cause swelling in the subtemporal region.

75

A   **F.**   In the first decade usually between ages 4 and 9 years. However the first episode may occur before age 2 years.

B   **F.**   Before age 5 years the normal tube is shorter and lies in a horizontal plane. This position detracts from the efficiency of muscles responsible for opening it. However in cleft palate cases additional anatomical defects of the eustachian tube account for the high prevalence of SOM.

C   **T.**   Due not only to physical blockage of the eustachian tube but also reduced tubal patency consequent upon an ascending salpingitis.

D   **T.**   Although the 'hydrops ex vacuo' probably plays some role. Evidence for the infective theory includes histopathological changes in glandular structures, isolation of viruses and bacteria and the high levels of IgA, IgG, lysozyme and protein in the effusion.

E   **T.**

76 Diagnosis and management of secretory otitis media
A   Varying head posture may alter the degree of deafness.
B   Pain is an uncommon feature.
C   A mobile eardrum excludes the diagnosis.
D   Cortical mastoidectomy may be necessary.
E   Chronic suppurative otitis media with cholesteatoma may be a
    late sequela.

77 Late sequelae of otitis media
A   Middle ear atelectasis is usually sited in the posterior half of the
    ear drum and may be reversed by ventilation.
B   Adhesive otitis media can be satisfactorily managed by division
    of fibrous bands and insertion of silastic sheeting.
C   The commonest site of intratympanic tympanosclerosis is the
    stapedius tendon.
D   Dry perforations of the pars flaccida are present in about 60%
    of cases of middle ear tympanosclerosis.
E   Attic tympanosclerosis may result in the 'fixed malleus
    syndrome'.

78 Tuberculous otitis media is
A   Usually painless.
B   Associated with multiple perforations of the pars tensa.
C   Occasionally heralded by a mastoid complication such as facial
    paralysis.
D   Possibly contracted by aspiration of milk via the eustachian
    tube.
E   Caused by treponema pallidum.

76

A   **T.**   Particularly if the middle ear fluid is thin. Hearing is best in bed.

B   **T.**   More likely to occur in acute secretory otitis media caused by flying or diving with an upper respiratory tract infection.

C   **F.**   Although mobility is usually absent an early or resolving effusion may have a mobile eardrum.

D   **T.**   Certain cases of secretory otitis media resistant to conventional treatment may have a co-existing secretory mastoiditis.

E   **T.**   Prolonged negative middle ear pressure predisposes to retraction pockets with accumulation of keratin and eventual cholesteatomatous chronic suppurative otitis media.

77

A   **T.**   Employing a combination of correcting nasal pathology and the insertion of long term ventilation tubes.

B   **F.**   Surgery is usually fruitless due to recurrent formation of adhesions and the risk of sensorineural deafness with ossicular reconstruction. The provision of a hearing aid is frequently the best management.

C   **F.**   The stapes–oval window region followed by the subfallopian and upper promontory sites.

D   **F.**   The perforations are almost exclusively confined to the pars tensa.

E   **T.**

78

A   **T.**

B   **T.**   May eventually coalesce to produce a single large defect. Pale granulations are frequently present.

C   **T.**   Also a cold subperiosteal abscess, labyrinthine fistula and tuberculous meningitis. Particularly in young patients.

D   **T.**   Cow's milk infected by bovine tuberculosis in pre-pasteurization days. Infection secondary to pulmonary tuberculosis is the usual cause nowadays.

E   **F.**   Caused by mycobacterium tuberculosis. The treponeme is the infective organism of syphilis.

79 Malignant tumours of the middle ear cleft

A Adenocarcinoma is the commonest histological type.
B Squamous carcinoma is usually associated with chronic otitis media.
C Intense pain is caused by meningeal involvement.
D Adenocarcinoma is radiosensitive and so surgery is reserved for residual or recurrent disease.
E Radical mastoidectomy is usually performed prior to radiotherapy.

80 Paragangliomas of the temporal bone

A Are more aggressive histologically than glomus tumours.
B May present with involvement of the 9th, 10th and 11th cranial nerves.
C Are more common in males.
D With massive intracranial extension are best treated with radiotherapy.
E May occur concurrently with a carotid body tumour.

81 Osseous disorders of the temporal bone

A Monostotic fibrous dysplasia is more common than the polyostotic type.
B Osteitis deformans has a rare tendency to sarcomatous change.
C Eosinophilic granuloma produces punched out lesions seen on plain X-rays.
D Osteopetrosis may present as recurring facial palsies.

79

A **F.**   Squamous carcinoma is. Adenocarcinoma is very rare and is usually due to direct extension of an adenocarcinoma of the external canal or deep lobe of the parotid.

B **T.**   Chronic infection probably causes squamous metaplasia. There is usually a very long history of CSOM. Many cases occur in chronically infected mastoidectomy cavities.

C **T.**   Pain, either its appearance or increase is a suspicious symptom in a chronic suppurative otitis media.

D **F.**   Adenocarcinoma is radioresistant. Radical surgery offers only hope of cure.

E **T.**   Allows an appreciation of the extent of disease, drainage, relief of pain and sepsis. The cavity can be more easily reviewed post-operatively and post-irradiation.

80

A **F.**   The terms are synonymous. Aggressiveness refers to clinical behaviour of a tumour rather than histology.

B **T.**   The so called 'jugular foramen syndrome', which may occur in glomus jugulare tumours.

C **F.**   Over 70% of cases are female.

D **T.**   Although surgery may be feasible the morbidity is considerable together with the risk of operative mortality. Radiotherapy can prevent progression for several years.

E **T.**   Paraganglionic tissue is also found in the turbinates, vagal bodies, larynx and aorta. All can give rise to paragangliomas.

81

A **T.**   Radiotherapy should be avoided as it predisposes to malignant change.

B **T.**   Usual sites of Paget's disease in the temporal bone are the cochlea and internal auditory canal. Can cause severe sensorineural deafness.

C **T.**   Conductive loss is due to ossicular involvement.

D **T.**   Behaves like Bell's palsy but each successive attack leaves a progressive residual weakness.

E **F.**   Very rare. It is usually preceded by a history of trauma.

82 Pathology of otosclerosis
A   Mature lamellar bone is removed and replaced by unorganized woven bone.
B   The commonest site is in the posterior promontory in the region of the fossula post fenestram.
C   Alpha-1-antitrypsin appears to play a role.
D   A type 4 otosclerotic footplate can be scored, fractured and removed.
E   Schwartze's sign indicates previous otitis media.

83 Patients with otosclerosis
A   Are commonly of negroid race.
B   May notice an onset or increase of deafness during pregnancy.
C   Without a family history may represent new mutations.
D   Have a female to male ratio of 2:1.
E   First have symptoms between 45 and 55 years in 70% of cases.

82
A   **T.**   The latter is of greater thickness, cellularity and vascularity. Hence the more apt descriptive term used by Europeans 'otospongiosis'.

B   **F.**   85% of cases occur anterior to the oval window in the fissula ante fenestram. This is a site of unossified bone.

C   **T.**   A dysequilibrium of the enzymes trypsin and alpha-1-antitrypsin in the cochlear may be a cause of 'cochlear otosclerosis' which is frequently associated with stapedial otosclerosis.

D   **F.**   Type 4 is obliterative with exostoses completely occluding the oval window and spreading to the crura. It requires a drill out or even an old fashioned fenestration procedure.

E   **F.**   It is a pink tinge (flamingo pink) that may be visualized on the promontory if the eardrum is thin. Occurs in rapidly progressive otosclerosis. Represents the highly vascular bone of the promontory seen through a thin tympanic membrane.

83
A   **F.**   It is rare in mongoloid and negroid man. Most patients are caucasian.

B   **T.**   Particularly about term. Thyrotoxicosis or onset of the menopause may also increase otosclerotic deafness. Probably related to the hormonal milieu and high metabolic activity.

C   **T.**   However, isolated cases may be a misdiagnosis or relatives may have histological otosclerosis without otological features.

D   **T.**

E   **F.**   90% of cases seen are between 15 and 45 years peaking in the third decade.

84 Diagnosis of otosclerosis
A   Paracusis Willisi may be present.
B   Notches at 1000 Hz and 50 Hz are seen on pure tone audiometric thresholds with air conduction.
C   Tympanometry is of little value.
D   Vertigo is invariably due to a labyrinthine hydrops.
E   Differential diagnosis from congenital footplate fixation is difficult as the conductive hearing loss is also progressive.

85 Treatment of otosclerosis
A   Sodium fluoride therapy is employed in pure cochlear otosclerosis.
B   Hearing aids halt the progression of otosclerosis.
C   Surgery is not usually indicated in unilateral ears with a normal contralateral ear.
D   Sensorineural losses may be encountered as late as 10 years after stapedectomy.
E   Fluorides may be administered safely during pregnancy.

86 During stapedectomy
A   Perilymph flooding may be due to an abnormally patent cochlear aqueduct.
B   A floating footplate is most likely to occur in a thick type 1 footplate.
C   The facial nerve presents no problems if it is in an intact fallopian canal.
D   Obliterative otosclerosis should be suspected if the preoperative compliance value is less than 0.2 ml air.
E   A persistent stapedial artery is encountered in about 30 cases per 1000 stapedectomies.

84

A **T.**   The phenomenon of hearing better in a background of noise.

B **F.**   Notches are seen on bone conduction . Carhart's notch at 2000 Hz is most common although other notches occur.

C **F.**   It can differentiate middle ear pathologies that mimic otosclerosis (ossicular discontinuity, fixed malleus/incus, etc.); the measure of compliance gives an indication as to the type of footplate likely to be encountered during surgery.

D **F.**   Usually due to changes in head posture. Hydrops may occur but is rare.

E **F.**   In congenital footplate fixation the hearing loss is frequently noted from early childhood and is non-progressive.

85

A **T.**   Although not all otologists agree that this form of otosclerosis exists. A skeletal survey to detect evidence of fluorosis is required every 2 years.

B **F.**   Utter nonsense. Hearing aids provide amplification. Aids with or without tinnitus maskers may be indicated.

C **T.**   In such cases surgery should be avoided. However if a hearing aid is refused or unhelpful and the preoperative speech discrimination is good, surgery may be contemplated. Successful surgery does allow the bonus of binaural hearing and sound localization.

D **T.**   Just one of many arguments against second side stapedectomy.

E **F.**

86

A **T.**   Prior to placing the prosthesis the flood may be controlled by inserting a spinal drain, parenteral mannitol and raising the head.

B **F.**   Usually the uniformly thick type 2 footplate. It is possible to get a satisfactory result by placing the prosthesis onto the floater if it cannot be easily delivered.

C **F.**   The canal itself may bulge down obscuring the oval window.

D **T.**

E **F.**   About 2–3/1000 stapedectomies.

87 Complications of stapedectomy
A   A divided chorda tympani always produces a loss or alteration of taste.
B   Balancing and labyrinthine exercises are useful in the early postoperative period.
C   Conductive hearing loss may be due to incus dislocation.
D   An overlong piston is better than one that is short.
E   Incus tip necrosis is the most frequent cause of recurrent conductive deafness.

88 Perilymph fistulae following stapedectomy
A   Inadequate closure of the fenestrated footplate is a cause.
B   The vein and polythene strut is the most frequent prosthesis involved.
C   Fluctuating hearing loss is a cardinal sign of a large fistula.
D   Tinnitus and hearing loss are usually improved if closure is successful.
E   The Fraser test may be positive.

87

A **F.** There may be no subjective complaints.

B **F.** Avoid all strain and sudden head movements. Flying, travelling by underground tube and sneezing with nose and/or mouth closed should be avoided. Cawthorne–Cooksey exercises may be helpful in cases of labyrinthine damage by hastening adaptation.

C **T.**

D **F.** The former is worse due to the high risk of early and late perilymph fistulae and subsequent sensorineural losses. The latter produce only a mechanical failure leading to persistent conductive hearing loss.

E **F.** A slipped prosthesis is the usual culprit, with a conductive hearing loss of about 60 dB and high compliance values.

88

A **T.** Usually fat or formalin free gelfoam is used. Vein or perichondrium can be used to bridge the fenestra. Stapedotomy appears to decrease the risk and does not require additional techniques.

B **T.** The sharp polythene tube pierces the vein membrane and enters the vestibule.

C **F.** Depends on the size of the fistula. Small fistulae are more likely to exhibit this sign, presumably because the leak is intermittent. Frequently the loss is of rapid onset and non-fluctuating.

D **F.** Vertigo is helped, hearing loss may be improved if repair is affected early (usually not the case) but tinnitus is rarely ameliorated. The tendency is for the diagnosis to be considered too late for effective action.

E **T.** The test is positive if after 20 min with the affected ear uppermost there is an improvement in the pure tone and/or speech audiometry. The pathophysiological basis is an air bubble in the cochlea causing a 'cochlear-conductive' hearing loss.

89 Van der Hoeve de Kleyn syndrome
A   Microscopic fractures with subsequent healing is the probable cause of stapedo-vestibular fixation.
B   Deafness does not occur without evidence of fractures.
C   Compliance values are low.
D   Stapedectomy is usually deferred until several years after spontaneous fractures have ceased.
E   Amelogenesis imperfecta may be associated.

90 In late syphilis in the temporal bone
A   Cochlear duct hydrops is a very common feature.
B   Hennebert's sign may be positive.
C   Steroids may improve the hearing deficit.
D   Interstitial keratitis may have occurred several years previously.
E   Tullio phenomena may be a symptom.

91 Congenital deafness
A   Rubella is an infrequent prenatal cause of sensorineural deafness.
B   A white forelock and heterochromia iridium may be associated.
C   Screening tests can only be reliably performed after 12 months of age.
D   A high tone loss is characteristic of cases caused by rhesus incompatibility.
E   Electric response audiometry is not particularly useful in assessing auditory function.

89

A **T.**

B **F.**   Deafness or deafness and blue sclerae can occur without fractures.

C **F.**   Usually very high despite ossicular fixation. Probably due to abnormal collagen causing excessive laxity of the ear drum.

D **T.**   The results are not as successful as in otosclerosis. There is a greater risk of a floating footplate and the bone is usually thick and vascular causing excessive haemorrhage.

E **T.**   In about 15% of cases. There is irregular dentine formation with yellow, opaque, irregular teeth.

90

A **T.**   Also involves the saccule and utricle. Sudden total or profound hearing loss may be due to rupture of the cochlear duct.

B **T.**   A fistula sign with an intact drum and no middle ear disease. Pathophysiologically due to energy transmission via the stapes footplate directly onto a distended saccule.

C **T.**   Should be given in combination with an appropriate antitreponemal agent such as benzylpenicillin.

D **T.**

E **T.**   A transient vertigo with nystagmus on sudden noise stimulation. Cause same as (B) above.

91

A **F.**   It is still a common prenatal cause but becoming less so. In the USA, a policy of vaccination of all children aims to greatly reduce the pool of infection in the community and hence cut the incidence of congenital rubella.

B **T.**   Waardenburg syndrome. Also includes features of a broad nasal bridge and lateral displacement of the medial canthi.

C **F.**   Should be conducted as early as possible.

D **T.**

E **F.**   Can provide very reliable objective measurement of thresholds in very young children. It will allow differentiation of those suffering from neurological disorders (mental deficiency, dyslexia) but whose hearing thresholds are normal.

92 Temporal bone fractures

A   About 80% are longitudinally placed.
B   The sensorineural hearing loss associated with longitudinal fractures does not recover.
C   Dysequilibrium may be caused by physical fatigue.
D   Facial paralysis is seen in about 50% of transverse fractures.
E   Cawthorne–Cooksey exercises may expedite vestibular compensation.

93 In closed head injuries without fracture

A   Hearing loss, if present, is most profound at 4000 Hz.
B   The most common vestibular symptom is positional vertigo.
C   Unilateral canal paresis is common.
D   Latent nystagmus may be revealed by removal of optic fixation.
E   Rapid acceleration may cause cochlear vestibular damage.

94 Inner ear barotrauma

A   A Valsalva manoeuvre, during a deep sea dive, in the presence of a locked eustachian tube may cause labyrinthine window rupture.
B   Decompression sickness is best treated by giving an oxygen–helium breathing mixture.
C   Patients with a short wide cochlear aqueduct are more prone to problems.
D   A previous stapedectomy reduces the risk of damage during flying.
E   Unilateral labyrinthine failure can be caused by changing from an oxygen–helium gas mix to compressed air at the start of decompression.

92

A	**T.**	
B	**F.**	It may do if the fracture has not transgressed the otic capsule. Commonly there is a conductive loss due to damage of middle ear structures.
C	**T.**	In unilateral vestibular failure the subsequent compensation may breakdown if other sources of sensory information are excluded. e.g. failing eyesight, fatigue, illness and drugs.
D	**T.**	
E	**T.**	

93

A	**T.**	Is usually bilateral.
B	**T.**	Of the benign paroxysmal variety. Perilymph fistulae due to labyrinthine membrane rupture may also be present.
C	**T.**	Occurring in about 60% of ears.
D	**T.**	
E	**T.**	Because of the relative inertia of the brain and membranous labyrinth in relation to the skull.

94

A	**T.**	Any diver with persistent giddiness or sensorineural deafness should be suspected of having a labyrinthine membrane rupture.
B	**F.**	Recompression is essential. This prevents gas bubbles within the inner ear.
C	**T.**	The infantile aqueduct is only 3.5 mm long and of relatively wide bore. This may persist into adulthood. It is unable to smooth out fluctuations in pressure differentials between the CSF and perilymph.
D	**F.**	The reverse is true.
E	**T.**	Gas bubbles are believed to form at the middle ear/ inner ear interface.

95 Excessive sound stimulation of the ear
A May cause transitory residual masking.
B A long lasting temporary threshold shift (TTS) recovers within 16 h.
C Can produce an acoustic notch at 6000 Hz.
D A short, intense single noise exposure may lead to permanent perceptive deafness.
E Can evoke the Tullio phenomenon only with an intact and mobile middle ear mechanism.

96 Infrasound
A Is easily detected by the human ear.
B Occurs in high speed automobiles particularly if the windows are open.
C May induce nystagmus.
D Could have caused the destruction of the 'Walls of Jericho'.
E Can be recorded on a normal tape-recorder.

97 Hearing conservation programmes in industry
A A sound profile of the potentially hazardous area is essential.
B Temporary threshold shifts do not adversely affect audiometric testing.
C The most effective hearing protector is the ear muff.
D Hearing protection need not be worn continuously in a high risk zone.
E Observation booths may be a practical solution.

95

A   **T.**   Transitory residual masking is a physiological adaptive phenomenon. A loud sound (up to 90 dB) elevates the threshold for an identical frequency presented immediately after. Frequencies above and below are affected to a lesser degree. Rapid exponential recovery occurs, within O.5 s for sounds up to 70 dB.

B   **F.**   Long lasting TTS are of greater than 16 h duration and merge imperceptibly with permanent threshold shifts.

C   **T.**   However a 4000 Hz dip is most commonly seen in practice. 6000 Hz is not a frequency that is tested on routine audiometry, but in some cases a 6000 Hz loss may occur earlier than the classical 4000 Hz dip.

D   **T.**   Termed 'Acoustic Trauma'.

E   **T.**   The term applied to noise induced vertigo. Probably due to excessive medial displacement of the stapes causing contact with a dilated saccule.

96

A   **F.**   By definition, infrasound is below the lower frequency limit of hearing. The ear is a very poor detector of sounds below 16 Hz.

B   **T.**   This accounts for some of the unpleasant sensations of light headedness and nausea that may be experienced.

C   **T.**   Probably by the Tullio phenomenon principle.

D   **T.**   If the correct resonant frequency had been emitted by the trumpets.

E   **F.**   Requires an FM (frequency modulation) tape recorder.

97

A   **T.**   That is, measurements of noise levels at various points.

B   **F.**   As the shift may be as high as 30 dB sufficient time between noise exposure and testing should be allowed to minimize this problem.

C   **T.**   If properly fitted can theoretically attenuate up to 50 dB in the higher frequencies.

D   **F.**   Non-adherence even for as little as a few minutes considerably reduces the value of protective measures.

E   **T.**   These separate the operative from the sound source.

98 Otitic blast injury
    A   Is an example of stimulation damage.
    B   Produces damage to the ear drum during the initial positive
          pressure wave.
    C   The extent of damage to the inner ear is reduced by an
          accompanying rupture of the ear drum.
    D   Only infrequently produces tinnitus.
    E   Does not produce vestibular symptoms.

99 Labyrinthine window rupture
    A   A preceding history of trauma can always be elicited.
    B   The round window is more frequently affected than the oval
          window.
    C   Symptoms and audiometry may be similar to Menière's disease.
    D   A rupture is usually visualized under high magnification.
    E   Surgical closure improves the hearing in over 60% of cases.

100 Otitic labyrinthitis
    A   Is most commonly due to surgical trauma such as
          stapedectomy or mastoidectomy.
    B   May be produced by a pathological fistula.
    C   Can occur after an acute viral illness.
    D   May result in ossification of the auditory nerve.
    E   Can not occur by direct spread of middle ear infection via the
          labyrinthine window membranes since they are impermeable.

98

A **T.**   Similar to a slap with the flat of the hand to the external ear.

B **T.**   This lasts about 5 ms and produces a pressure of several thousands of pounds per square inch.

C **F.**   Long lasting high-tone perceptive deafness is frequently seen despite the presence of perforations.

D **F.**   Tinnitus is an invariable symptom.

E **F.**   Benign paroxysmal positional vertigo may be observed. Perilymph fistulae may also occur.

99

A **F.**   Although trauma is frequent (closed head injury, barotrauma) even slight exertion (lifting, sneezing, coitus) causing a rise in intracranial pressure may be the initiating factor. Spontaneous ruptures can also occur.

B **F.**   The reverse is true and occasionally both are involved.

C **T.**   In such cases a positive Fraser's test is highly suggestive of a perilymph leak.

D **F.**   Frequently its presence can only be inferred from the leakage of fluid. Normal seepage of tissue fluid or injected infiltration solution can mislead the surgeon. Jugular pressure, head down position and Valsalva under GA are manoeuvres which can be employed if there is no obvious leak, but have the disadvantage that venous oozing may be induced.

E **F.**   Hearing is improved in about 30%. Vestibular symptoms are relieved in about 80%. Tinnitus is rarely improved.

100

A **F.**   Chronic suppurative otitis media with extension is the commonest aetiological factor.

B **T.**   Usually due to erosion of the lateral semicircular canal but occasionally the promontory. If the membranous labyrinth is not breached this condition may only produce symptoms during the fistula test. Terms employed for this condition include paralabyrinthitis, perilabyrinthitis and circumscribed labyrinthitis.

C **T.**   Acute coryza (adenovirus type 3): mumps, measles, herpes zoster or may accompany myringitis bullosa haemorrhagica.

D **F.**   There may be sclerosis (labyrinthitis ossificans) in both the vestibule and cochlea as the end result of suppurative labyrinthitis.

E **F.**   Can occur in acute infections.

101 In circumscribed labyrinthitis
- A   Symptoms may be precipitated by auricular movement.
- B   Autoinflation is the most effective method of eliciting the fistula sign.
- C   In a weakly positive fistula sign nystagmus without vertigo is elicited.
- D   If caused by atticoantral CSOM is an indication for conservative management.
- E   The hearing deficit will not recover.

102 In syphilitic labyrinthitis
- A   The highest incidence occurs in the late stage of neurosyphilis.
- B   The fluorescent treponemal antibody absorbed test (FTA-ABS) is the least reliable serological test.
- C   Microscopic endolymphatic hydrops is a common feature.
- D   Vestibular reactions are completely lost.
- E   Fibrous bands may connect the medial surface of the stapes footplate to the membranous labyrinth.

103 Pathophysiology of Menière's Disease
- A   Sympathetic overactivity may play a role.
- B   There is gross dilatation of the scala vestibuli.
- C   Fibrous bands may connect the footplate to the distended saccule.
- D   Ruptures of the membranous labyrinth have been postulated as the cause of acute attacks.
- E   Sodium and potassium levels in the endolymph are grossly abnormal.

101

A	T.	Also by head movement, sneezing and coughing.
B	F.	Pneumomassage with Siegle's speculum or rhythmical tragal pressure may elicit the nystagmus and vertigo.
C	F.	Nystagmus absent but vertigo present.
D	F.	Some form of mastoid exploration will be required. Exteriorization is essential.
E	F.	May improve.

102

A	T.	About 80%. Incidence of inner ear involvement is about 18% in congenital and 25% in secondary syphilis.
B	F.	It is positive in 100% of acquired and 98% of congenital cases.
C	T.	Clinically the symptoms and signs closely mimic Menière's disease.
D	F.	Maybe, but patient may display vestibular paradox, i.e. absent caloric stimulation but elicitable rotational reactions.
E	T.	This or erosion of the bony labyrinth may account for the occasional presence of Hennebert's signs (positive fistula sign without middle ear disease) and Tullio phenomenon (vertigo and nystagmus induced by noise).

103

A	T.	By producing vasospasm in the microcirculation leading to sensory impairment and interference with the secretion of endolymph. Sympathectomy may produce dramatic relief of vertigo. Hence local anaesthesia injection in the region of the cervical sympathetic may abort an acute Menières attack.
B	F.	The scala media (cochlear duct) and saccule are dilated.
C	T.	
D	T.	Rupture and subsequent healing may explain the exacerbations and remissions that characterize Menière's disease.
E	F.	Most studies show that levels of these cations are relatively normal.

104 Clinical manifestations of Menière's disease
  A   Vertiginous attacks characteristically occur without warning.
  B   Utricular crises are common.
  C   Horizontal nystagmus is absent during an acute crisis.
  D   Migrainous headaches may be associated with vertiginous
      attacks.
  E   Diplacusis is a suggestive diagnostic feature.

105 Cogan's disease is characterized by
  A   Audiovestibular symptoms and interstitial keratitis.
  B   Vertigo without hearing loss or tinnitus.
  C   An improvement in hearing and tinnitus with the onset of
      vertigo.
  D   Copious otorrhoea.
  E   Radiological expansion of the internal auditory canal.

106 Investigation of Menière's disease
  A   A normal caloric response excludes the diagnosis.
  B   The glycerol dehydration test is especially useful in patients with
      near normal hearing.
  C   Speech audiometry is helpful in differentiation between sensory
      and neural deafness.
  D   Electrocochleography may reveal changes in the unaffected
      ear.
  E   Vestibular aqueduct tomography is essential.

104

A **F.**   About 50% of patients have prodromal symptoms, e.g. muffled hearing, heaviness or pressure in the ear. Some attacks start with loudening of tinnitus, or a change in its character, often described as 'roaring'.

B **F.**   Also known as 'drop attacks', very uncommon. These occur without warning.

C **F.**   Always present and its direction may vary between and during attacks. Between attacks it may be elicited only by ENG with abolition of optic fixation.

D **T.**   Some claim the association in as many as 20% of cases.

E **T.**   A sound of a given frequency is perceived to be a different pitch in each ear.

105

A **T.**   The keratitis is non-syphilitic.

B **F.**   This combination of symptoms occur in vestibular neuronitis.

C **F.**   These are the symptoms of Lermoyez's syndrome, a rare variant of Menière's disease.

D **F.**

E **F.**

106

A **F.**   Caloric responses are usually paretic, a directional preponderance to either side may be seen. Normal responses can occur during the remission phase.

B **F.**   The test depends upon the demonstration of an improvement in hearing thresholds. If they are nearly normal it would be difficult to improve them further. It is most useful in patients with fluctuating hearing loss. If in remission the test is unreliable.

C **T.**   Speech discrimination in cochlear deafness is usually better than in neural deafness with similar pure tone thresholds.

D **T.**   Classically shows a large summating potential and an abnormal cochlear microphonic. The sensitivity of the test is enhanced by administration of acetazolamide (hydration). Electrical changes are reduced with glycerol (dehydration). In unilateral cases the test may reveal the contralateral ear to be affected.

E **F.**   A research investigation. If performed the aqueduct is shown to be narrowed.

107 Medical management of Menière's disease
A   There is a sound pathophysiological basis for prescribing a salt free diet.
B   Nicotinic acid does not produce an increase in cochlear blood flow.
C   Diuretic therapy improves the long term course of the disease.
D   Cinnarizine is a useful vestibular sedative.
E   Streptomycin is useful as it has a purely vestibulotoxic effect.

108 Surgical management of Menière's disease
A   Vertiginous symptoms are least likely to be ameliorated.
B   Georges Portmann was the first to perform a saccus endolymphaticus drainage procedure.
C   An endolymphatic perilymphatic shunt can be created by cochleostomy.
D   A middle fossa approach should be utilized for division of the vestibular nerve.
E   A membranous labyrinthectomy is generally performed by a postaural approach opening the lateral semicircular canal.

109 Pathology of presbyacusis
A   Sensory presbyacusis is characterized by atrophy of the organ of Corti in the basal turn of the cochlea.
B   A reduction in the number of cochlear spiral ganglion cells to 2000 produces a minimal effect on speech reception.
C   A flat pure tone audiometric curve is usually seen in cochlear conductive presbyacusis.
D   The middle ear function plays a significant role in the audiometric changes.
E   The rate of degeneration has an inherited predisposition.

107

A	**F.**	Although prescribed by some otologists. A few patients appear to benefit.
B	**T.**	Although frequently prescribed. Betahistine has revealed some benefit.
C	**F.**	Diuretics are used to reproduce the improvement seen by the osmotic/diuretic effect of glycerol but it does not alter the long term prognosis.
D	**T.**	It has both phenothiazine (antiemetic) and antihistamine properties.
E	**F.**	There is a danger of cochlear injury, particularly in the presence of inadequate renal function.

108

A	**F.**	Most surgical procedures are designed to relieve vertigo. They may also prevent further hearing losses of a permanent nature.
B	**T.**	In 1927. It would appear that the sac merely requires to be exposed, without incision and drainage, to produce benefit.
C	**T.**	Using an angled pick, inserted via the round window the scala tympani (perilymph) and scala media (endolymph) are connected by puncturing the basilar membrane. Devised by H.F. Schuknecht. The high risk of sensorineural hearing loss has discouraged its use.
D	**F.**	A posterior fossa approach is possible. If there is no hearing a translabyrinthine neurectomy is feasible.
E	**F.**	Although this approach is described the Schuknecht procedure is preferable. This is a permeatal approach with avulsion of the utricle after elevating the stapes footplate and placing a sucker through the round window membrane and instillation of 90% alcohol.

109

A	**T.**	Hence the abrupt high tone loss. Speech discrimination remains satisfactory late in the process.
B	**F.**	There is a severe loss of speech discrimination as found in neural presbyacusis. The ganglion cell population is normally 30 000.
C	**F.**	Strial atrophy produces a flat curve with a reasonable speech discrimination score. Cochlear conductive presbyacusis, probably due to changes in the motion mechanics of the basilar membrane, produces a descending audiometric pattern for bone conduction.
D	**F.**	Although thickening of the eardrum and ankylosis and laxity of ossicular articulation has been reported there is only a minimal effect on hearing thresholds.
E	**T.**	

110 Management of presbyacusis
A   Sibilant and fricative consonants are well heard.
B   The patient is more likely to understand the raised loud voice.
C   Electronic hearing aids are the mainstay of treatment.
D   Lip reading and auditory training are useful adjuncts.
E   Amplification within the dynamic range provides better voice intelligibility.

111 The ototoxic effects of
A   Streptomycin are predominantly vestibulotoxic.
B   Neomycin may be delayed weeks or months following administration.
C   Salicylates are irreversible.
D   Anticonvulsant drugs can cause toxic effects on the vestibular system.
E   Diuretics are usually permanent.

112 Objective tinnitus
A   Is more common than subjective tinnitus.
B   Palatal myoclonus is the commonest cause.
C   Intraaural muscles usually produce subjective tinnitus.
D   Head and neck auscultation is mandatory.
E   Costen's syndrome may be the aetiology.

110

A	**F.**	Badly heard as the high frequency tones are usually lost early in the process.
B	**F.**	Increased intensity may produce recruitment. The voice should be clearly articulated, normal in character and close to the patient's ear.
C	**T.**	Particularly those with low tone cut and automatic volume control facilities.
D	**T.**	But not easily mastered by the elderly.
E	**T.**	But amplification to levels above the patient's loudness discomfort level results in distortion and reduced intelligibility.

111

A	**T.**	But with high doses and prolonged treatment cochleotoxic effects are seen. The drug has been used in bilateral Menière's disease to ablate vestibular function.
B	**T.**	Also with dihydrostreptomycin. All the aminoglycosides may exhibit this feature. Neomycin has a predominantly cochleotoxic effect.
C	**F.**	Tinnitus and/or hearing loss are usually reversible. Aetiology is a probable vasoconstriction of the cochlear microcirculation. Prostaglandins are implicated.
D	**T.**	Phenytoin in particular may produce a 'posterior fossa syndrome'. Cerebellar degeneration has been shown with chronic administration. Ethosuximide has similar vestibulotoxic side effects.
E	**F.**	Both ethacrynic acid and frusemide usually produce a temporary sensorineural deafness on intravenous administration. Rarely it may be permanent.

112

A	**F.**	Objective tinnitus is a relative rarity.
B	**T.**	May be visualized, palpated and auscultated.
C	**F.**	Myoclonic contractions of the stapedius and tensor tympani may cause clicking tinnitus.
D	**T.**	Either with a meatal stethoscope, cochlear microphone or routine stethoscope. Vascular skull abnormalities may produce a pulsatile tinnitus.
E	**T.**	Sounds transmitted to the external meatus from an abnormal temporomandibular joint.

113 Subjective tinnitus

A   Is a frequent occurrence in severe congenital deafness.
B   If tonal in quality may reveal a dip on the pure-tone audiogram at the frequency of the tinnitus.
C   Is not masked by hearing aids.
D   Can be suppressed by electrical stimulation.
E   May be made worse with ablative surgery.

113

A	**F.**	Very rare. Auditory experience appears to be a prerequisite for developing tinnitus.
B	**T.**	Due either to a masking effect or an actual reduction of the threshold.
C	**F.**	Usually very valuable. Can be combined with a tinnitus masker. Only very high tonal tinnitus is difficult to mask.
D	**T.**	Employing direct current, which produces suppression only whilst flowing; alternating current may additionally produce residual inhibition after stimulation has ceased.
E	**T.**	

SECTION 2
NOSE AND SINUSES

114 Blood supply of the nose

A   Branches of both internal and external carotid arteries supply the nasal mucosa.

B   The maxillary artery provides the major blood supply to the nasal fossa.

C   Little's area is supplied by branches of the greater palatine, sphenopalatine, posterior ethmoidal and superior labial arteries.

D   Venous drainage occurs into the superior sagittal sinus via the foramen caecum.

E   Sympathetic motor fibres controlling the mucosal vessels run in the Vidian nerve.

115 Nasal anatomy

A   The cell bodies of olfactory neurones lie in the nasal mucosa.

B   The greater palatine nerve supplies most of the inferior turbinate with common sensation.

C   The posterior lateral nasal nerves are branches of the posterior ethmoidal nerve.

D   Lymph from the anterior part of the nose drains to the submental nodes.

E   The posterior part of the nasal cavity drains to the retropharyngeal and upper deep cervical lymph nodes.

116 Examination of the nose and sinuses

A   The superior turbinate is easily seen in the child by turning up the tip of the nose with the thumb.

B   Application of vasoconstrictor solutions is contraindicated in the examination of the nose.

C   The best view of the eustachian tube orifices is obtained by a fibreoptic nasolaryngoscope passed through the mouth.

D   Transillumination is a useful physical sign in the examination of the paranasal sinuses.

E   Ultrasound scanning is the most accurate method of diagnosing maxillary sinusitis.

114

A **T.** The maxillary artery is an end branch of the external carotid; the internal carotid supplies blood to the superior part of the nose via the anterior and posterior ethmoidal branches of its ophthalmic branch.

B **T.** 90% of the nasal mucosa is supplied from the maxillary artery, and transantral ligation is an effective treatment for severe epistaxis.

C **F.** Anterior ethmoidal.

D **T.** The foramen caecum lies in front of the crista galli and transmits an emissary vein from the nose to the superior sagittal sinus.

E **T.** Both sympathetic and parasympathetic fibres run in the Vidian nerve, from the internal carotid plexus and greater superficial petrosal nerve respectively. The main effect of Vidian neurectomy, however, is to abolish parasympathetic overactivity.

115

A **T.** They are bipolar cells with non-medullated central processes terminating in the olfactory bulb.

B **T.** The lateral branch of the anterior ethmoidal nerve supplies the remainder.

C **F.** They are branches of the sphenopalatine (pterygopalatine) ganglion.

D **F.** Submandibular nodes.

E **T.** The fact that retropharyngeal nodes are often involved in spread of posterior nasal and nasopharyngeal tumours makes radical neck dissection a poor treatment, since the intervening retropharyngeal nodes cannot be excised.

116

A **F.** Only the inferior and middle turbinates will be seen. This is the correct technique for examining the nose in a child.

B **F.** Vasoconstrictors are very useful in this situation.

C **F.** The eustachian tube orifices are best seen with a mirror. Where this is not possible, the fibreoptic nasolaryngoscope is passed along the nose.

D **F.** Transillumination is only rarely of any help, and is not routinely performed.

E **F.** Antroscopy is the most accurate method. Proof puncture and antral lavage was the 'gold standard', but it is possible to fail to obtain pus when it is excessively thick or when loculation has occurred. X-rays are about 85% accurate. Coronal CT scanning provides more precise information but is expensive and not widely available.

117 Sinus X-rays
    A   The maxillary antrum is best seen in an occipitomental view.
    B   The frontal sinuses are well shown in an occipitofrontal view.
    C   The sphenoidal sinus is obscured by the temporomandibular joint on the standard lateral view.
    D   The posterior ethmoidal sinuses are seen in a submentovertical view.
    E   CT scanning is of no more value than plain X-rays in neoplasms of the nose and sinuses.

118 Operations on the nose and sinuses
    A   External approaches to the sinuses are in general safer than intranasal.
    B   The area below and lateral to the attachment of the middle turbinate is the 'danger area' in intranasal surgery.
    C   The outer wall of the ethmoidal labyrinth is relatively thick and unlikely to be penetrated except by excessive force.
    D   If meningitis follows intranasal surgery, the cribriform plate must have been penetrated.
    E   The optic nerve is too far back to be injured during intranasal surgery.

119 Antral washouts
    A   Are usually performed through the middle meatus.
    B   Are virtually free of complications.
    C   May require a second cannula if the ostium is blocked.
    D   May be done as a diagnostic or therapeutic manoeuvre.
    E   The opening into the sinus is permanent.

117

A **T.**   In an OMV the head is tilted backward by about 20 degrees, to lift the maxillary antrum clear of the dense shadow of the petrous temporal bone.

B **T.**

C **F.**   The sphenoidal sinus is well shown on a standard lateral view.

D **T.**

E **F.**   CT scanning offers significant improvements over plain films. Lesions are shown at an earlier stage, their site can be more accurately assessed and bone destruction seen at an earlier stage. Coronal scans, where available, may provide more reliable information on the important question of intracranial extension of disease.

118

A **T.**   Because of the improved direct visual access.

B **F.**   The danger area is above and lateral to the attachment of the middle turbinate.

C **F.**   The lamina papyracea is literally paper thin.

D **F.**   Infection can spread via perineural lymphatics of the olfactory nerve filaments, and via the roof of the ethmoids.

E **F.**   The optic nerve is at risk, particularly posteriorly.

119

A **F.**   The inferior meatus is more commonly used. The middle meatus carries a risk of subsequent stenosis of the ostium, and the orbit is more easily entered.

B **F.**   The list of complications includes haemorrhage, blindness, meningitis and air embolism, among others.

C **T.**

D **T.**

E **F.**   Even the large defect created by a formal antrostomy tends to close over.

120 Sinus operations
A   The Caldwell Luc operation includes routine division of the descending palatine artery.
B   The anterior ethmoidal air cells are best approached by the transantral (Jannsen Horgan) route.
C   In the Howarth external fronto-ethmoidectomy, the frontonasal duct is removed.
D   The sphenoidal sinus can be approached by the intranasal, transantral, external ethmoidectomy, transpalatal and trans-septal routes.
E   The ethmoidal sinuses can be widely exposed in lateral rhinotomy.

121 Nasal respiration
A   Neonates are obligate nose breathers.
B   Nasal breathing reflexly stops during swallowing.
C   The anterior end of the inferior turbinate is important in regulating inspiratory airflow.
D   Expiratory air currents are determined solely by the state of the posterior choanae.
E   Eddy currents under the middle turbinate help provide conditioned air around the sinus ostia.

122 The mucociliary 'conveyor belt' of the upper respiratory tract
A   The cilia beat 100 times a second.
B   The movement directs the mucus to the anterior nares.
C   Lysozymes are produced by bacteria and act to paralyse cilia.
D   A deviated nasal septum can produce localized drying with ciliary stasis, crusting and secondary infection.
E   Ephedrine 0.5% nose drops cause ciliary damage.

123 Anosmia
A   Must be bilateral before it is noticeable.
B   Is often described as loss of taste.
C   Can be tested by simple objective methods.
D   May be due to a brain tumour.
E   Usually recovers after skull fracture, beginning about 12 months after the injury.

120

A **F.**   The opening of the nasal antrostomy into the inferior meatus should not extend too far posteriorly, or the descending branches of the sphenopalatine and greater palatine arteries will be damaged, with severe haemorrhage.

B **F.**   The transantral approach gives poor exposure of the anterior ethmoidal cells, they are best approached externally.

C **T.**   Together with removal of the floor of the frontal sinus and the anterior ethmoidal cells, to create a wide passage into the middle meatus.

D **T.**

E **T.**

121

A **T.**   Congenital bilateral choanal atresia presents as a neonate who fails to breathe until he becomes distressed, then is able to breathe through the mouth while crying. When crying ceases the cycle repeats itself. Emergency treatment is to provide an oral airway.

B **T.**

C **T.**

D **F.**

E **T.**

122

A **F.**   10 times a second.

B **F.**   The mucus is directed to the nasopharynx.

C **F.**   Lysozymes are protective bacteriolytic enzymes produced by the nasal mucosa.

D **T.**   Drying may be localized, or generalized due to constant exposure to dry air, e.g. central heating.

E **F.**   However, prolonged use of any vasoconstrictor will cause rebound congestion and may result in chronic hypertrophic rhinitis (rhinitis medicamentosa).

123

A **T.**

B **T.**   Flavours are mainly perceived by olfaction.

C **F.**   Clinical test solutions of, e.g. lemon, cloves, require subjective responses and are unreliable. Objective testing—electro-olfactography—is complicated and imperfectly developed.

D **T.**   Particularly frontal lobe lesions.

E **F.**   Where anosmia follows skull fracture, recovery is unlikely if it has not begun within 3 months.

124 Disorders of smell
  A   Hyposmia can be caused by vasomotor rhinitis in the absence of mechanical obstruction.
  B   Where influenza causes a peripheral olfactory neuritis, the loss of smell is usually permanent.
  C   Cacosmia may be due to a foreign body in the nose.
  D   Temporal lobe epilepsy may cause olfactory hallucinations.
  E   Ammonia is used to stimulate the olfactory nerve in suspected malingerers.

125 Cleft lip and cleft palate
  A   The cleft lip results from failure of fusion of the maxillary process with the median nasal process.
  B   Flattening of the nostril is a feature.
  C   The nasal septum may be abnormally thick.
  D   The deformities result from teratogenic or genetic factors operating in the second month of foetal life.
  E   Bifid uvula is a minor form.

126 Congenital nasal malformations
  A   A midline dermoid cyst should be distinguished from a meningocoele at operation.
  B   A fistula is often present with dermoid cysts.
  C   Aplasia of the maxillary sinus is as common as aplasia of the frontal sinus.
  D   Exorbitism is a feature of Crouzon's syndrome.
  E   Atresia of the anterior nares is common in Negroes.

127 Congenital choanal atresia
  A   Is most commonly a membranous closure.
  B   Is most commonly bilateral.
  C   Occurs more often in females.
  D   If unilateral tends to present late with persistent watery rhinorrhea.
  E   Bilateral cases may be fatal.

128 Management of maxillofacial injuries
  A   The first consideration is to look for signs of shock.
  B   The patient should be positioned supine.
  C   X-ray is the most useful diagnostic manoeuvre.
  D   Nasal obstruction indicates septal dislocation or haematoma.
  E   Asch's forceps are used to correct septal deformity.

124

A **T.**
B **T.**
C **T.**   Cacosmia is the perception of a bad smell due to an intrinsic cause.
D **T.**
E **F.**   Ammonia stimulates the trigeminal nerve. It is used to test for psychogenic causes.

125

A **T.**
B **T.**   Especially in cases of bilateral cleft lip.
C **T.**
D **T.**
E **T.**

126

A **F.**   The distinction should be made preoperatively.
B **T.**
C **F.**   Failure of pneumatization is not uncommon in the frontal sinus, but rare in the maxillary.
D **T.**   Crouzon's syndrome is a form of craniofacial dysostosis, characterized by calvarial deformity, mid-face hypoplasia and exorbitism.
E **F.**   It is rare in all races.

127

A **F.**   Most are bony.
B **F.**   Unilateral is commoner, 60% of cases.
C **T.**   Ratio 2:1.
D **F.**   Late presentation is the rule, but the nasal discharge is thick and tenacious.
E **T.**   The neonate is an obligate nasal breather. Failure to provide an oral airway can result in death from asphyxia.

128

A **F.**   The first consideration is the airway.
B **F.**   The patient should be in the recovery position.
C **F.**   The diagnosis can usually be made clinically. X-rays are mainly of medicolegal importance.
D **T.**

129 Middle third facial fractures
A   Le Fort I (Guerin) involves the orbit.
B   Malocclusion is common.
C   Trismus is due to associated temporomandibular joint dislocation.
D   Epiphora indicates involvement of the nasolacrimal duct.
E   An opaque antrum on X-ray is an indication for antral puncture and lavage.

130 Blowout fracture of the orbit
A   Is caused by excessive force blowing the nose.
B   The eyeball herniates into the antrum.
C   The patient is unable to look down.
D   Treatment should be delayed until oedema has settled if the forced duction test shows limitation of movement.
E   Silastic sheeting is a suitable material for repair of the orbital floor.

131 Fractures involving the frontal or ethmoidal sinuses
A   CSF rhinorrhoea implies a dural tear.
B   Nose blowing may cause an intracranial aerocoele.
C   Systemic antibiotics are routinely given to prevent meningitis.
D   If the posterior wall of the frontal sinus alone is involved, and there is no aerocoele, early repair is unnecessary.
E   A fascial graft may be used to repair a dural tear.

132 Cerebrospinal fluid rhinorrhoea
A   The usual symptom is clear watery fluid dripping from the nose.
B   The fluid contains glucose.
C   The site of the leak is determined by clinical examination.
D   Initial treatment is to pack the nose with BIPP.
E   A lumboperitoneal shunt should be considered before resorting to craniotomy.

129

A	**F.**	The Le Fort I fracture passes below the orbit. Types II and III do involve the orbit.
B	**T.**	This is one of the main diagnostic features. It requires skilled treatment by an oral surgeon.
C	**F.**	Trismus is due to a combination of malocclusion and soft tissue swelling.
D	**T.**	
E	**F.**	An opaque antrum is due to blood, and does not require lavage.

130

A	**F.**	The cause is a backward blow on the eyeball.
B	**F.**	Orbital fat, with or without the inferior rectus muscle, herniates into the antrum.
C	**F.**	Upward gaze is limited. Other eye movements are usually unaffected.
D	**F.**	Treatment should be as soon as possible if diplopia is to be avoided.
E	**T.**	

131

A	**T.**	
B	**T.**	This is commonest if the lamina papyracea is fractured.
C	**T.**	Penicillin and sulphadimidine are the traditional choice.
D	**T.**	The indication for early fascial repair is intracranial aerocoele. Persistent CSF leak may require late repair.
E	**T.**	Other materials are now being used, e.g. collagen felt and tissue glue.

132

A	**T.**	Some cases present with meningitis.
B	**T.**	Tested by dextrostix.
C	**F.**	The site of the leak may be very difficult to demonstrate. Methods used include X-ray (shows fractures and bone erosion) CT scanning with or without metrizamide cisternography, and injection of radioactive tracer into the CSF, collected onto cotton wool pledgets in the nose.
D	**F.**	This would be extremely dangerous and could lead to meningitis. Treatment initially consists of prophylactic antibiotics, with strict avoidance of nose-blowing or any local interference.
E	**T.**	

133 Oro-antral fistula
A   Dental extraction is the usual cause of the alveolar type.
B   Regurgitation of food into the nose is a symptom.
C   Maxillary sinusitis frequently ensues.
D   Intranasal antrostomy is part of the treatment.
E   The rim of a sublabial fistula should be excised.

134 Bullet wounds in the head and neck region
A   High velocity missile wounds are less likely to be contaminated than low velocity.
B   Damage far from the path of the bullet may be caused by a travelling shock wave.
C   The first principle of treatment is to excise devitalized tissue.
D   Primary closure is contraindicated.
E   Fixation of facial fractures is unnecessary.

135 Sinus barotrauma
A   Is due to excessively high pressure in the sinus.
B   Is more likely to occur in the presence of an upper respiratory tract infection.
C   Pain is usually felt during descent.
D   Submucosal haemorrhage is a pathological feature.
E   Decongestant nasal drops are helpful prophylactically.

136 Nasal septal deformities
A   May be caused by birth trauma.
B   Deviated septum is associated with high arched palate.
C   A spur predisposes to epistaxes.
D   Submucous resection is the treatment of choice in children.
E   The perichondrial layer should be conserved in SMR.

133

A   **T.**   Other causes are erosion by malignancy and penetrating wounds. Caldwell Luc and similar operations may cause a sublabial fistula.

B   **T.**   Regurgitation of air and fluid is commoner.

C   **T.**   The infection tends to produce particularly foul smelling pus with dental cases.

D   **T.**   To allow drainage into the nose. A general principle of treatment for any fistula is to provide proximal drainage.

E   **T.**   The mucosal edges are then undercut and sutured.

134

A   **F.**   A high velocity missile causes a large cavity to form, the vacuum sucks in dirt and organisms from the skin.

B   **T.**   The intima of the carotid artery may be lifted up in this way.

C   **F.**   Devitalized tissue should be excised, but the first principle of treatment is to safeguard the airway.

D   **F.**   Primary closure can be undertaken in this region because of the excellent blood supply.

E   **F.**   Fixation may be essential.

135

A   **F.**   Low pressure.

B   **T.**   Because the sinus ostium is then more likely to be obstructed, preventing pressure equalization.

C   **T.**

D   **T.**   Earlier changes are mucosal congestion, inflammation, oedema, and haemorrhage. Submucosal haemorrhage occurs in severe cases.

E   **T.**

136

A   **T.**   This is however a rare cause. Most are due to trauma later in life.

B   **T.**   The congenital high arched palate leaves less room for the vertical height of the septum, which tends to buckle.

C   **T.**   Bleeding occurs from vessels over its sharp convex surface.

D   **F.**   Children are treated either by expectant management, waiting until they are around 16 years, or by conservative septoplasty. Standard SMR is likely to produce deformity of growth.

E   **T.**   The operation should really be termed a submucoperichondrial resection.

137 Septal haematoma
A   Is usually traumatic in origin.
B   May be due to a blood dyscrasia.
C   Unilateral nasal obstruction is the commonest symptom.
D   Is likely to resolve spontaneously without complication.
E   Treatment is conservative unless an abscess develops.

138 Septal abscess
A   Is always secondary to a septal haematoma.
B   Pain is localized to the tip of the nose.
C   Systemic symptoms are unusual.
D   A septal perforation may ensue.
E   Initial treatment consists of incision and drainage plus systemic antibiotics.

139 Septal perforation
A   Most cases are due to nose-picking, syphilis or cocaine abuse.
B   Chromic acid is a recognized industrial cause.
C   Large perforations characteristically cause a whistling noise.
D   The cartilaginous septum is most commonly involved, except in syphilitic cases, when it is the bony septum.
E   Surgical repair is usually advisable because of the danger of severe epistaxes.

140 Foreign bodies in the nose
A   Usually present in adult life.
B   Epistaxis is the commonest clinical feature.
C   Non-organic materials cause more tissue reaction than organic.
D   A bead should be removed with non-toothed dissecting forceps.
E   General anaesthetic is often required in children.

137

A	**T.**	Trauma may be external or surgical.
B	**T.**	
C	**F.**	Bilateral obstruction.
D	**F.**	Septal abscess and subsequent cartilage necrosis are likely. In the absence of infection, permanent gross thickening of the septum is likely.
E	**F.**	The haematoma should be evacuated, provision for drainage made, and nasal splints and/or packs inserted to prevent a further accumulation. Systemic antibiotics are prescribed to prevent secondary infection.

138

A	**F.**	It may also follow nasal furuncle, or occur spontaneously in the course of childhood exanthemata.
B	**F.**	Severe generalized headache is the commonest type of pain associated. The nose is locally tender.
C	**F.**	The patient is generally unwell with fever.
D	**T.**	Cartilage necrosis may also occur with subsequent nasal collapse. Rarely, cavernous sinus thrombosis or meningitis ensues.
E	**T.**	

139

A	**F.**	The majority of cases are traumatic in origin, usually following submucous resection.
B	**T.**	
C	**F.**	Small perforations cause whistling.
D	**T.**	
E	**F.**	Conservative treatment is usual, with e.g. glucose and glycerin drops to prevent crusting. Epistaxis from septal perforation is usually minor, and follows separation of crusts. A silastic 'button' can be used. Many cases are asymptomatic and require no treatment.

140

A	**F.**	Much commoner in children.
B	**F.**	Either present acutely as a known foreign body, or with a chronic unilateral nasal discharge.
C	**F.**	Organic materials cause severe mucosal inflammation.
D	**F.**	Should be removed with a blunt hook. Forceps are likely to push the foreign body deeper into the nose.
E	**T.**	No attempt should be made to remove a foreign body in an uncooperative child.

141 Rhinolith
A   Is a stony hard nose due to infiltration with tumour.
B   Can be formed from an organized blood clot.
C   Is characterized by extreme pain.
D   Can often be detected using a probe.
E   Is radio-opaque.

142 Inflammation of the external nose
A   Furunculosis arises in a pilosebaceous follicle in the vestibule.
B   Cavernous sinus thrombosis is a complication.
C   Painful fissures occur in chronic vestibulitis.
D   Erysipelas is an acute spreading staphylococcal dermatitis.
E   Acne rosacea may progress to rhinophyma.

143 Acute infective rhinitis
A   Is most commonly caused by the rhinovirus.
B   Green discharge indicates secondary bacterial infection.
C   Otitis media is a common complication in children.
D   Vasoconstrictor nose drops should not be used.
E   Vaccination provides effective protection.

144 Chronic non-specific rhinitis
A   Aetiological factors include atmospheric pollution and excessive dryness.
B   A deviated nasal septum predisposes.
C   The goblet cells increase while ciliated cells are lost from the epithelium.
D   Nasal obstruction commonly alternates from side to side.
E   Inferior turbinectomy is the treatment of choice.

141

A **F.** A rhinolith is a concretion of calcium and magnesium salts which builds up over many years around a foreign body in the nasal fossa. It can also form around inspissated mucus or blood clot (endogenous rhinolith).

B **T.**

C **F.** Unilateral nasal obstruction and discharge are the characteristic symptoms. Some rhinoliths go unrecognized for many years.

D **T.** A grating sensation is felt.

E **T.** Because of the calcification.

142

A **T.**

B **T.**

C **T.**

D **F.** Streptococcal.

E **T.**

143

A **T.**

B **T.** Organisms include *Strep. pneumoniae, Staph. aureus, H. influenzae and Klebsiella.*

C **T.** The middle ear mucosa is an extension of the upper respiratory tract.

D **F.** They provide effective symptomatic relief of nasal obstruction, and may prevent the complication of sinusitis. However they should not be used for longer than a week.

E **F.** This is because there are so many different viruses which cause the condition (at least 200) it is not feasible to vaccinate against all of them. Influenza vaccines are used to protect patients at special risk, e.g. chronic bronchitics, but they only protect against a specific strain of influenza virus.

144

A **T.** The condition is multifactorial in origin.

B **T.** By causing localized areas of dryness and crusting, or by interfering with normal drainage.

C **T.** Cf. chronic bronchitis.

D **T.** An exaggeration of the normal nasal cycle. When lying down, the dependent nostril is blocked.

E **F.** Surgical treatment is reserved for cases where pathological changes are irreversible and/or medical treatment has failed.

145 Chronic hypertrophic rhinitis
A   Can be caused by abuse of vasoconstrictor drops ('rhinitis
    medicamentosa').
B   The mucosa of the inferior turbinates is particularly affected.
C   A mulberry turbinate may be seen prolapsing through the
    nostril.
D   Fibrosis causing lymphatic obstruction may lead to polyp
    formation.
E   Treatment consists of oral antihistamines and local injection of
    sclerosants.

146 Atrophic rhinitis
A   The patient suffers from cacosmia.
B   The primary form is commonest in young women.
C   Syphilis should be excluded.
D   Local treatment is with glucose 25% in glycerin drops.
E   Surgery to narrow the nasal airways may be effective.

147 Wegener's granulomatosis
A   Affects the nose, lungs and kidney.
B   Is fatal without treatment.
C   The pathological lesion is similar to polyarteritis nodosa.
D   Treatment is by local radiotherapy.
E   Combination steroid and cytotoxic therapy improves survival
    over steroid alone.

145

A   **T.**   It may also be simply an advanced case of chronic non-specific rhinitis.

B   **T.**

C   **F.**   The mulberry turbinate is the hypertrophied posterior end, and is seen occupying the choana on mirror examination of the nasopharynx.

D   **T.**   Although polyps are more commonly found in allergic and vasomotor rhinitis.

E   **F.**   Treatment consists of stopping any predisposing factors e.g. vasoconstrictor abuse, smoking, alcohol abuse, attention to sinus infection, local treatment with steroid spray, followed by surgical removal of chronically hypertrophied mucosa, straightening of septal deviations and polypectomy.

146

A   **F.**   Cacosmia is the perception of a bad smell in the nose due to an intrinsic cause. Although patients with atrophic rhinitis have a foul smell in the nose, they are themselves anosmic.

B   **T.**

C   **T.**

D   **T.**

E   **T.**

147

A   **T.**   Other regions may also be involved, e.g. ear, pharynx.

B   **T.**   Sometimes in a very short space of time—24 h in fulminant cases. Death is usually from renal failure.

C   **T.**   Giant cells are also seen in the granulomata. However histological confirmation of the disease may be difficult; frequently a clinical decision has to be made to start treatment.

D   **F.**   Radiotherapy is used in Stewart's 'granuloma', which is in fact a low grade lymphoma.

E   **T.**   Azathioprine and cyclophosphamide are used, and have revolutionized the prognosis.

148 Syphilis and the nose
  A   'Snuffles' affects infants aged 2–5 years with congenital syphilis.
  B   Nasal chancre is associated with painful submaxillary lymphadenopathy.
  C   Secondary syphilis may masquerade as a persistent coryza.
  D   A gumma is the commonest nasal manifestation of syphilis.
  E   Serological tests are unlikely to be positive in tertiary syphilis.

149 Nasal lupus vulgaris
  A   Is a tuberculous infection of the skin.
  B   The source is frequently pulmonary TB in a family member.
  C   'Apple jelly nodules' are seen histologically.
  D   The cartilaginous septum may perforate.
  E   Antituberculous drugs promote rapid healing without deformity.

150 Chronic specific rhinitis
  A   Sarcoidosis usually presents as an atrophic ulcer.
  B   Yaws is the commonest cause of a runny nose in Jamaica.
  C   Leprosy causes excruciatingly painful ulceration.
  D   Rhinosporidiosis presents as a bleeding raspberry-like polyp.
  E   Nasopharyngeal Leishmaniasis is transmitted by the South American sandfly.

151 Acute infective sinusitis
  A   Is usually caused by a preceding coryza.
  B   Can follow barotrauma.
  C   If secondary to dental infection, the causative organism is likely to be *Haemophilus influenza*.
  D   There is reduced mucosal glandular secretion initially.
  E   An empyema is a collection of seromucinous fluid in the sinus.

148

A **F.** Snuffles affects the neonate, up to around 3 months. It can cause major difficulties with feeding.

B **F.** The lymphadenopathy is painless.

C **T.** Other manifestations should be looked for, e.g. snail track ulcers, rash, generalized lymphadenopathy.

D **T.** It usually occurs in the bony septum, but any part of the nose may be affected.

E **F.** Approximately 90% will be positive. Serology is usually negative in primary syphilis.

149

A **T.**

B **T.**

C **F.** Apple jelly nodules are seen clinically, by pressing on the affected skin with a glass slide. The histological appearances are typical of tuberculosis elsewhere, namely caseating granulomata with giant cell formation.

D **T.**

E **F.** Antituberculous drugs will arrest the course of the disease, but healing is by fibrosis and deformities will occur. Of course, any destruction of tissue that has already taken place cannot be reversed by drug treatment. Plastic reconstructive procedures will often be required.

150

A **F.** Nasal sarcoid usually presents as nodules or crusting on the septum, vestibule or anterior ends of inferior turbinates. It may also present as a lupus pernio. Widespread distribution is characteristic.

B **F.** Although Yaws is common in Jamaica, it rarely affects the nose.

C **F.** Lepromatous ulceration is painless because the peripheral nerves are destroyed.

D **T.**

E **T.**

151

A **T.**

B **T.**

C **F.** Anaerobic organisms are characteristic of dental infection. *H. influenzae* causes epidemics of sinusitis, particularly in children.

D **F.** There is hypersecretion.

E **F.** Contains infected mucopus.

152 Acute infective sinusitis
A   Pain is limited to the area overlying the affected sinus.
B   Oedema of the overlying tissues is commoner in children.
C   Mucopurulent nasal discharge is necessary to make the diagnosis.
D   Decongestant nose drops are used to provide 'medical drainage'.
E   An antibiotic solution should be instilled into the sinus cavity during antral lavage.

153 Chronic non-specific sinusitis
A   May be due to an unresolved attack of acute sinusitis.
B   Vasomotor rhinitis is the aetiological factor in two-thirds of cases.
C   Multiple small abscesses in the thickened mucosa are a recognised pathological feature.
D   Bacteriology usually reveals pure cultures of streptococci.
E   Postnasal drip is a *sine qua non* for the diagnosis.

154 Mixed infective and vasomotor chronic sinusitis
A   Eosinophils and polymorphonucleocytes are found in the discharge.
B   The frontal sinus is most commonly affected.
C   Polyps are often found and may block the sinus ostia.
D   Topical steroid therapy should be avoided because of the danger of uncontrolled infection.
E   A radical operation offers a good prospect of permanent cure.

152

A	**F.**	Pain from sinusitis can radiate widely. Tenderness is usually localized over the affected sinus.
B	**T.**	Swelling of the cheek in maxillary sinusitis, and of the orbit in ethmoidal sinusitis.
C	**F.**	The discharge is only present if the sinus is draining ('open sinusitis'). A closed sinusitis can cause severe symptoms, but there is no mucopurulent discharge because the ostium is blocked.
D	**T.**	Vasoconstriction of the congested nasal mucosa around the sinus ostia promotes drainage.
E	**F.**	Systemic antibiotics are given. Washouts are performed with either saline or water.

153

A	**T.**	
B	**T.**	
C	**T.**	The pathological appearances are variable, even within the individual patient. Polyps, atrophic mucosa, fibrosis, epithelial metaplasia, abscesses, cysts and granulations all occur.
D	**F.**	Mixed growth is usual. Anaerobes are common. *Strep. pneumoniae* and gram-negative bacilli often coexist.
E	**F.**	

154

A	**T.**	Eosinophils are especially prominent when there is an allergic component, polymorphonucleocytes when infection predominates.
B	**F.**	Maxillary and ethmoidal sinuses are most commonly affected.
C	**T.**	
D	**F.**	Topical steroid therapy is one of the most effective forms of treatment and has very few side effects. Antibiotics are indicated in the presence of active infection.
E	**F.**	The condition is chronic and unlikely to be cured. Surgery has a role in providing an adequate airway when this cannot be achieved medically, in the removal of irreversibly diseased mucosa, and provision of drainage for obstructed sinuses.

155 Acute maxillary sinusitis
A   The infection is of dental origin in 1% of cases.
B   Tenderness is usually localized over the sinus.
C   X-rays are of no value in the acute phase.
D   Antral washouts should be performed as soon as possible, to establish the diagnosis and commence treatment.
E   Toothache precedes sinusitis in all cases of apical abscess.

156 Acute frontal sinusitis
A   The frontal sinus is usually affected alone.
B   Pain is typically worse in the morning.
C   Discharge is seen in the inferior meatus, where the frontonasal duct opens.
D   Treatment is to cannulate the frontonasal duct.
E   Trephining the orbital roof should be avoided because of the danger of spreading infection to the eye.

157 Acute sphenoidal sinusitis
A   Is not uncommon.
B   The posterior ethmoidal cells are involved in most cases.
C   Pain may simulate acute mastoiditis.
D   Discharge is seen at the back of the nose.
E   The sinus can be punctured and washed out transnasally.

158 Treatment of chronic maxillary sinusitis
A   Medical treatment is useless; surgery is nearly always required.
B   Antral washouts should be performed daily for 3 weeks in the first instance.
C   Polyps in the sinus can be removed most effectively via intranasal antrostomy.
D   Caldwell–Luc operation involves enlarging the natural ostium to allow free drainage.
E   A sublabial antrostomy is contraindicated in the presence of irreversible pathological change in the mucosa.

155

A	**F.**	Dental infection causes around 10% of cases.
B	**T.**	Although the pain can radiate widely, the tenderness is usually localized.
C	**F.**	X-rays are the main diagnostic investigation.
D	**F.**	Antibiotics and nasal decongestants should be given first. If the response is unsatisfactory, antral washouts should be performed.
E	**F.**	A dead tooth with apical abscess can be painless.

156

A	**F.**	The anterior ethmoidal and maxillary sinuses are usually affected as well.
B	**T.**	
C	**F.**	The frontonasal duct opens into the middle meatus.
D	**F.**	Cannulation of the frontonasal duct is difficult and will probably damage the duct. Treatment consists of systemic antibiotics, local decongestants, treatment of concurrent maxillary sinusitis, and, in severe cases, trephine of the floor of the frontal sinus via the orbital roof. A plastic tube can then be left in place for irrigation until the infection is under control.
E	**F.**	See above.

157

A	**F.**	It is rare.
B	**T.**	Most commonly as part of a pansinusitis.
C	**T.**	Pain may radiate anywhere in the head.
D	**T.**	
E	**T.**	Rarely performed.

158

A	**F.**	Medical treatment has improved, particularly with antibiotics and local steroids. Surgery is now required much less frequently than in the past.
B	**F.**	Very few patients would tolerate this medieval regime.
C	**F.**	Open operation such as a Caldwell–Luc is the most effective method. Endoscopic surgery can also be used to remove polypi.
D	**F.**	The antrostomy is made into the inferior meatus.
E	**F.**	This is the main indication for sublabial antrostomy (Caldwell–Luc operation).

159 Treatment of chronic frontal sinusitis
A   Catheterization of the frontonasal duct should precede more radical operations.
B   The Howarth operation combines treatment of frontal and maxillary sinuses.
C   A drainage tube is left in the nose for several weeks after the Howarth operation.
D   Obliteration of the sinus is an alternative to a drainage procedure.
E   An osteoplastic flap is hinged superiorly.

160 Aetiology of sinusitis in children
A   Antibody deficiency is a common cause.
B   Dietary deficiency and poor social conditions are contributory.
C   Bacteriology usually shows a pure growth of *Haemophilus influenzae* in chronic cases.
D   Childhood exanthemata may initiate chronic sinusitis.
E   Kartagener's syndrome consists of sinusitis, bronchitis, and congenital cyanotic heart disease.

161 Sinusitis in children
A   The frontal sinus is poorly developed before the 5th year.
B   In acute sinusitis, oedema of the cheeks and eyelids is commoner in children than adults.
C   Pain is the principal clinical feature of chronic sinusitis in children.
D   Chronic ethmoidal sinusitis should be treated by external ethmoidectomy.
E   Adenoidectomy may improve the outlook in chronic maxillary sinusitis.

159

A   **F.**   Catheterization of the frontonasal duct is ineffective and may result in subsequent stenosis, making drainage worse.

B   **F.**   The Howarth procedure comprises fronto-ethmoidectomy via a curved incision around the medial border of the orbit. Patterson's approach, where the incision is below the orbital margin, is used for combined access to maxillary and ethmoidal sinuses.

C   **T.**   The objective is to form a wide drainage channel from the frontal and anterior ethmoidal cells into the middle meatus.

D   **T.**

E   **F.**   Inferiorly.

160

A   **F.**   Antibody deficiency is a rare cause.

B   **T.**

C   **F.**   Cultures are usually mixed in chronic cases. *H. influenzae* is often responsible for acute sinusitis.

D   **T.**

E   **F.**   Sinusitis, bronchiectasis and dextrocardia. The common defect is in ciliary structure. The fact that the kinocilium is affected results in loss of polarity in embryonic development and hence dextrocardia. The heart condition is asymptomatic.

161

A   **T.**

B   **T.**

C   **F.**   Pain is often absent. Nasal obstruction, mucopurulent rhinorrhoea, mouth breathing, snoring, coughing and ear problems are the main clinical features. Early morning vomiting may occur.

D   **F.**   Conservative management is preferred. Predisposing factors should be treated, e.g. allergy, and neighbouring infections controlled.

E   **T.**   Chronically infected and enlarged adenoids act as a source of infection and may obstruct normal drainage which is via the nasopharynx.

162 Spread of infection in suppurative sinusitis
  A   Osteitis occurs in compact bone.
  B   Osteomyelitis occurs in diploic bone.
  C   Meningitis usually arises via a septic thrombophlebitis.
  D   Lymphatic channels are involved in the formation of
      subperiosteal abscesses.
  E   Spread into the subarachnoid space can occur via the
      perineural space around the olfactory nerves.

163 Osteomyelitis of the frontal bone
  A   Is most frequently due to frontal sinusitis.
  B   Streptococci and staphylococci are the commonest bacteria
      responsible.
  C   The onset is usually acute with rigors or epileptic fits.
  D   Pott's puffy tumour is a malignant myxomatous degeneration.
  E   Intracranial complications are a remote possibility.

164 Osteomyelitis of the frontal bone
  A   X-rays do not show any bony abnormality until sequestration
      occurs.
  B   Antibiotic treatment is ineffective.
  C   The floor of the frontal sinus should be trephined in severe
      cases with sequestration and intracranial infection.
  D   Opening the anterior wall of the sinus is contraindicated.
  E   Where bone has to be removed in young patients, the defect
      may regenerate spontaneously.

165 Orbital complications of suppurative sinusitis
  A   All the paranasal sinuses border the orbit at some point.
  B   Orbital complications are most common in children.
  C   A subperiosteal abscess due to frontal sinusitis points
      anteriorly.
  D   Orbital cellulitis usually precedes abscess formation.
  E   Thrombophlebitis may result in cavernous sinus thrombosis.

162
  A **T.**
  B **T.**
  C **T.** Further spread causes intracranial venous sinus thrombosis, and extradural, subdural and brain abscesses. Distant venous spread may cause septicaemia and endocarditis.
  D **T.** The lymphatics accompany blood vessels through their bony foramina.
  E **T.**

163
  A **T.** Particularly where the sinus is operated on without antibiotic cover.
  B **T.** The streptococci may be anaerobic.
  C **F.** The onset is usually insidious, with dull local pain. Rigors and fits occur later, signifying septicaemia and intracranial spread respectively.
  D **F.** Pott's puffy tumour is an oedematous swelling of the soft tissues overlying the infected bone.
  E **F.** Extradural abscess is likely to follow unless treatment is prompt.

164
  A **F.** In the first week there will be no changes other than those of the frontal sinusitis or trauma. A loss of bone pattern then appears, followed by thinning, necrosis and sequestration.
  B **F.** High dose intravenous antibiotics are the mainstay of treatment.
  C **F.** This procedure would be inadequate for such cases. They would require more radical surgery.
  D **F.** The anterior wall of the sinus must be opened where sequestration has occurred, to remove the dead and infected bone.
  E **T.** However grafts will often be necessary.

165
  A **T.**
  B **T.** Usually due to ethmoidal infection.
  C **T.**
  D **T.**
  E **T.**

166 Orbital complications of suppurative sinusitis

A   Eye movements exacerbate the pain of orbital cellulitis.
B   Proptosis means that an abscess has formed.
C   The fundus in orbital cellulitis is pale because of compression of the ophthalmic artery.
D   A mucocoele can always be distinguished from an abscess by the sign of eggshell crackling.
E   A rapidly growing orbital tumour can simulate orbital cellulitis.

167 Intracranial complications of suppurative sinusitis

A   Frontal sinusitis is associated with frontal lobe abscess.
B   Ethmoidal sinusitis is associated with diffuse suppurative meningitis.
C   Sphenoidal sinusitis is associated with cavernous sinus thrombosis.
D   Maxillary sinusitis is particularly likely to cause intracranial complications.
E   Intracranial spread of infection may occur via the pterygoid venous plexus in maxillary sinusitis.

168 Secondary effects of suppurative sinusitis

A   Infection from the nasopharynx may cause laryngitis.
B   Sinus infection may cause chronic secretory otitis media.
C   Maxillary sinusitis is the cause of bronchiectasis.
D   Antral washouts should precede thoracic surgery where sinusitis and bronchiectasis coexist.
E   Successful treatment of chronic sinusitis may improve asthma.

166

A	**T.**	
B	**F.**	Proptosis simply means that the globe has been displaced forward. Any expanding mass in the orbit can do this.
C	**F.**	The fundus shows congestion because of venous compression.
D	**F.**	If the mucocoele has eroded the bone completely there will be no eggshell crackling.
E	**T.**	

167

A	**T.**	Extradural and subdural abscess, and thrombophlebitis of the sagittal sinus and cortical veins over the frontal lobe may also occur.
B	**T.**	The route of spread is usually via the roof of the ethmoidal labyrinth.
C	**T.**	Also with diffuse meningitis, and thrombophlebitis of other intracranial venous sinuses.
D	**F.**	
E	**T.**	However it occurs more often because of other paranasal sinus involvement concurrently with the maxillary sinusitis.

168

A	**T.**	A chronic postnasal drip of infected mucopus may cause lateral pharyngitis, tonsillitis and laryngitis.
B	**T.**	
C	**F.**	The two conditions are associated, and exacerbate one another, but the relationship is not causal. Some rare cases are due to a congenital defect in ciliary motility (Kartagener's syndrome), or abnormally viscid mucus secretion (cystic fibrosis); others may be due to the long term effects of damage to the respiratory tract sustained during a childhood attack of pertussis or measles.
D	**T.**	Sometimes more radical sinus surgery is indicated.
E	**T.**	Such treatment can sometimes allow the dose of steroids and bronchodilators to be reduced.

169 Transitional cell papilloma (Ringertz tumour)
A   Is usually indistinguishable from an allergic nasal polyp.
B   Most arise from the nasal septum.
C   May have areas of columnar and squamous epithelium.
D   Malignant transformation only occurs after irradiation.
E   Complete removal is the treatment of choice.

170 Benign tumours of the paranasal sinuses
A   Ivory osteoma of the frontal sinus is the commonest type.
B   The commonest presentation is headache due to pressure erosion of the anterior cranial fossa.
C   Mucocoele and ocular displacement are complications of frontal sinus osteoma.
D   Localized fibro-osseous dysplasia in children should be excised completely because of the danger of malignant change.
E   Hyperostosis frontalis interna is a cause of headache in elderly females.

171 Malignant tumours of the nose and paranasal sinuses
A   Squamous cell carcinoma is the commonest type.
B   Retropharyngeal and cervical lymph node metastases are common.
C   Adenoid cystic carcinoma is associated with woodworkers in the furniture industry.
D   An ameloblastoma is a rapidly growing, highly malignant tumour.
E   Burkitt's lymphoma is confined to African children.

169

   A   **F.**   Most will be unilateral, whereas allergic polyps are usually bilateral. The surface appearance is different, being grey and wrinkled or fleshy rather than the gelatinous appearance of a typical allergic polyp. However no gross appearance is diagnostic, and cases will be missed unless all polyps are sent for histology.

   B   **F.**   The majority arise from the lateral nasal wall, some from the antrum or ethmoidal sinuses.

   C   **T.**   The epithelium is grossly thickened and infolded, leading to the alternative pathological description of 'inverted papilloma'. Epithelial atypia is common, but the basement membrane remains intact.

   D   **F.**   There is an incidence of around 10% malignancy; there is dispute whether this is malignant transformation or whether the malignant tumours are malignant from the outset. Malignant behaviour may be early or delayed many years. Radiotherapy should not be given to non-malignant cases as prophylaxis.

   E   **T.**   This will usually require lateral rhinotomy.

170

   A   **T.**   Incidence up to 1% of skulls.

   B   **F.**   Commonest presentation is an incidental finding on X-ray.

   C   **T.**   Occur when the tumour obstructs the frontonasal duct or is large enough to expand into the orbit.

   D   **F.**   Malignant change is not a problem, unless the condition is unwisely treated with radiotherapy. A biopsy may be necessary to differentiate from a malignant tumour, but following this it is best left alone until growth has ceased, when cosmetic reduction can be undertaken. Earlier surgical intervention may be necessary if local complications ensue, such as a threat to vision from orbital involvement.

   E   **T.**

171

   A   **T.**   80% of malignant tumours. The majority are differentiated.

   B   **F.**   Metastases occur in about 5%. Failure to control local disease is the usual cause of death.

   C   **F.**   Adenocarcinoma.

   D   **F.**   It is slowly growing and relatively benign.

   E   **F.**   Cases have occurred elsewhere, including the USA, and in adults as well as children.

172 Malignant tumours of the paranasal sinuses
A   Ohngren's line extends from the lateral canthus to the symphysis menti.
B   Lederman's classification uses horizontal lines drawn through the superior and inferior orbital margins.
C   Pain is the earliest clinical feature.
D   Epiphora indicates involvement of the frontonasal duct.
E   Biopsy is usually unnecessary as the diagnosis can be made radiologically.

173 Treatment of malignant tumours of the paranasal sinuses
A   Sublabial antrostomy for biopsy is contraindicated because of the risk of tumour implantation.
B   If the tumour penetrates the cribriform plate it is inoperable.
C   Radical surgery followed by radiotherapy gives 5 year survival figures of 80% overall.
D   Orbital involvement is a contraindication to radical maxillectomy.
E   Cytotoxic drug treatment is the first line of management.

174 Pituitary tumours
A   Most pituitary tumours are malignant.
B   Acromegaly is usually due to an acidophil adenoma.
C   Cushing's syndrome can be treated by hypophysectomy.
D   Transphenoidal hypophysectomy is particularly suitable for suprasellar tumours.
E   The optic chiasma is at greater risk from transfrontal craniotomy than a transphenoidal approach.

172

A **F.** Ohngren's line extends from medial canthus to angle of jaw, dividing the maxillary antrum into inferomedial and superolateral halves. Tumours arising inferomedially tend to have a slightly better prognosis because they cause nasal symptoms earlier, can often be seen on examination of the nose, and total resection is more often feasible.

B **F.** The horizontal lines traverse orbital and antral floors, forming three regions—suprastructure, mesostructure and infrastrucure. In addition, vertical lines passing down from the medial orbital walls separate the nasal fossa and ethmoids from the antra. This system has the advantage of including the whole of the nose, upper and lower jaws, and all the sinuses.

C **F.** Pain is usually late, from involvement of the maxillary nerve, facial tissues or dura.

D **F.** Epiphora is due to nasolacrimal duct obstruction. Involvement of the frontonasal duct results in frontal sinusitis or occasionally a mucocoele.

E **F.** Biopsy is essential. It may be carried out via the nose, or a Caldwell–Luc may be necessary.

173

A **F.** This approach is used for biopsy. Any tissue implanted would be excised at maxillectomy.

B **F.** Craniofacial resections are increasingly carried out.

C **F.** Unlikely to exceed 35%.

D **F.** Orbital clearance is combined with radical maxillectomy in such cases.

E **F.** Cytotoxic chemotherapy is still confined to the role of adjuvant treatment. It is potentially dangerous and should only be carried out in specialized hospital units, preferably as part of a controlled trial since further information on efficacy is still required.

174

A **F.** Nearly all are benign.

B **T.** Modern cytohistochemical methods stain according to the hormone produced. Acromegalics produce excessive growth hormone.

C **T.** Provided it is due to an ACTH secreting pituitary tumour, rather than an adrenal tumour or a side effect of steroid therapy.

D **F.** A small suprasellar extension is not a contraindication, but large suprasellar lesions will need a craniotomy.

E **T.**

175 Maxillary cysts
A   A midline swelling in the palate is likely to be malignant.
B   A median alveolar cyst is of developmental origin.
C   A nasopalatine cyst arises from the incisive canal and can present either in the nose or on the palate.
D   A lateral alveolar cyst separates incisor from canine teeth, at the line of fusion between maxilla and premaxilla.
E   A naso-alveolar cyst usually presents as a loose tooth.

176 Cysts of dental origin
A   Primordial cysts are malignant.
B   A cyst of eruption arises over a tooth that has not erupted.
C   A tooth is usually inside a dentigerous (follicular) cyst.
D   Dental (radicular) cysts imply previous or current root infection.
E   A dental cyst may persist after root extraction.

177 Radiographic diagnosis of maxillary cysts
A   A clear outline is typical of developmental cysts.
B   Multiple cysts may be due to cherubism.
C   Hyperparathyroidism characteristically causes a single giant cyst with a sharply defined margin.
D   An osteoclastoma is usually radiolucent.
E   A myelomatous deposit is usually radio-opaque.

178 Odontogenic tumours
A   Arise solely from developing dental epithelium.
B   Are commonest in young adults and children.
C   An adamantinoma contains enamel.
D   A composite odontoma is so called because it incorporates more than one tooth.
E   An ameloblastoma is likely to metastasize widely.

179 Causes of epistaxis
A   Idiopathic bleeding from Little's area is commonest.
B   Digital trauma (nosepicking) is a common cause.
C   A septal spur predisposes.
D   Low atmospheric pressure and low humidity increase the incidence.
E   Venous hypertension is a factor in chronic bronchitics.

175

A	**F.**	It is likely to be of developmental origin.
B	**T.**	Lies between the upper central incisors.
C	**T.**	
D	**T.**	
E	**F.**	Usually presents as nasal obstruction, or external deformity with a wide nostril and loss of the nasolabial fold. It lies in the floor of the nose anteriorly and displaces the inferior turbinate upwards.

176

A	**F.**	A primordial cyst is formed from enamel organ epithelium before dental tissue.
B	**T.**	
C	**T.**	
D	**T.**	
E	**T.**	

177

A	**T.**	
B	**T.**	The cysts are symmetrically arranged, affecting both maxilla and mandible.
C	**F.**	Causes multiple poorly defined radiolucent areas, with alteration of normal bony trabeculation.
D	**T.**	
E	**F.**	Radiolucent with round 'punched out' appearance.

178

A	**F.**	May also arise from mesodermal elements.
B	**T.**	
C	**F.**	Now known as ameloblastoma, this locally invasive tumour probably arises from the epithelial debris of Malassez, which comprises remnants of the primary dental lamina.
D	**F.**	Because it is formed of more than one germinal layer—ectoderm and mesoderm.
E	**F.**	Locally malignant, cf. basal cell carcinoma.

179

A	**T.**	
B	**T.**	
C	**T.**	Also makes treatment difficult. Septal surgery may be required.
D	**T.**	Both factors operate together at altitude.
E	**T.**	

180 Sites of bleeding in epistaxis
A Little's area is the anterior end of the inferior turbinate.
B Kiesselbach's plexus is in the pterygopalatine fossa.
C Bilateral epistaxis implies bleeding from the nasopharynx.
D Bleeding above the level of the middle turbinate is likely to originate from the internal carotid artery.
E Bleeding from the middle meatus may be due to a tumour in the maxillary sinus.

181 Initial treatment of severe epistaxis
A The patient should be placed head down supine with a pillow under the shoulders.
B Trotter's method includes encouraging the patient to swallow the blood, to allay psychological stress and thereby reduce blood pressure.
C A postnasal pack should be considered when the haemoglobin falls below 10 g/litre.
D Epistaxis balloons should be inflated with sterile water.
E A central venous pressure line is mandatory.

182 Surgical intervention in epistaxis
A Failure to control bleeding by cautery or packing is an indication for examination under anaesthesia.
B Blood transfusion should not be undertaken unless the haemoglobin is below 10 g/dl.
C Transantral ligation of the maxillary artery is ineffective because of collateral circulation from the Circle of Willis.
D Ligation of the common carotid is a useful alternative to transantral maxillary ligation in the elderly patient.
E The anterior ethmoidal artery can be approached via a Howarth incision.

180
A	**F.**	Little's area is the anterior part of the septum.
B	**F.**	Kiesselbach's plexus is in Little's area.
C	**F.**	Bilateral epistaxis is commonly due to the original side being partially blocked by the patient or by clot; blood then passes behind the choana and down the opposite nasal fossa. Alternatively there may be more than one site, but bleeding from the nasopharynx is rare.
D	**T.**	From the anterior ethmoidal, a branch of the ophthalmic, supplied from the internal carotid.
E	**T.**	This is a rare cause.

181
A	**F.**	It is difficult to think of a worse position. The patient should be seated in a chair, leaning forward, breathing through the open mouth, and allowing blood to drip into a bowl. The anterior part of the nose is compressed between finger and thumb to put pressure on Little's area, which is the site of bleeding in 90% of cases. Ice packs can be applied to the forehead or bridge of the nose. An atmosphere of calm efficiency should prevail.
B	**F.**	Trotter's method is described above.
C	**F.**	A postnatal pack is used when an adequate anterior pack fails to control bleeding. A haemoglobin of 10 g/litre is not compatible with life (= 1 g/dl).
D	**F.**	Should be inflated with air, which conforms better and will not cause aspiration problems if it bursts.
E	**F.**	Rarely required unless complications are present.

182
A	**T.**	
B	**F.**	Blood transfusion is indicated for blood loss in excess of 10% of the circulating blood volume. After acute blood loss, the haemoglobin may remain normal for several hours until haemodilution occurs.
C	**F.**	Transantral ligation is an effective operation. Failure is due to technical deficiency or bleeding from the anterior ethmoidal artery.
D	**F.**	External carotid ligation is occasionally useful, as it is quick and can be performed under local anaesthetic if necessary. The problem of collateral circulation is less if it is tied distal to the lingual branch. Ligation of the common carotid would probably cause a stroke or death of the patient.
E	**T.**	

183 Epistaxis in hereditary haemorrhagic telangiectasia
A   Is rarely a significant problem.
B   Androgens are used in treatment.
C   Injection of sclerosants is usually curative.
D   Septodermoplasty involves excision of the septal mucosa and replacing it by a split skin graft.
E   Bleeding may occur lower down the gastrointestinal tract.

184 Vasomotor rhinitis
A   The nasal mucosa is hyper-reactive.
B   Parasympathetic over-activity is implicated.
C   Puberty may initiate the condition.
D   Symptoms are usually worse in pregnancy.
E   Rhinitis medicamentosa is due to Beta blockers.

185 Clinical features of vasomotor rhinitis include
A   Paroxysmal sneezing attacks.
B   Alternating intermittent bilateral nasal obstruction.
C   Thick green foul-smelling rhinorrhoea.
D   Nasal polyps.
E   Mulberry turbinates.

186 Medical treatment of vasomotor rhinitis
A   Precipitating factors should be identified and avoided if possible.
B   Antihistamines are especially useful for obstructive symptoms.
C   Topical steroids are the mainstay of medical treatment.
D   Vasoconstrictors should be administered systemically.
E   Epistaxis is a recognized side-effect of topical steroids.

183

A **F.** Bleeding is frequent and can be severe. No treatment is permanently effective; multiple blood transfusions and operations are often required.

B **F.** Oestrogens.

C **F**

D **T.** Effective for 2 or 3 years, then telangiectases recur on the grafted area.

E **T.** Can be fatal, despite control of nosebleeds.

184

A **T.** A wide range of trigger factors cause excessive secretion, sneezing and vasodilation, by non-allergic mechanisms.

B **T.**

C **T.** Presumably an endocrine effect.

D **T.**

E **F.** Beta blockers do cause nasal congestion in some patients, but rhinitis medicamentosa refers to chronic hypertrophic rhinitis with rebound congestion caused by excessive prolonged use of local sympathomimetic vasoconstrictor drops.

185

A **T.**

B **T.**

C **F.** This would suggest sinus infection or foreign body.

D **T.**

E **T.**

186

A **T.** Smoking and alcohol especially.

B **F.** Sometimes useful for sneezing and profuse watery rhinorrhoea.

C **T.** Either spray or drops.

D **F.** Can be dangerous; tachyphylaxis occurs limiting usefulness.

E **T.** A different formulation may help, e.g. changing from aerosol to aqueous beclomethasone.

187 Surgical treatment of vasomotor rhinitis
A   Is necessary in the majority of cases.
B   Headache is an indication for diathermy to the middle
turbinates.
C   Septal surgery may be helpful even if the cartilaginous deformity
is minor.
D   Reduction of the inferior turbinates is an out-patient procedure.
E   Long term cure is to be expected.

188 Aetiology of allergic rhinitis
A   It is often familial.
B   IgE is the reaginic antibody.
C   Co-existing asthma or eczema implies atopy.
D   Inhaled allergens are the commonest trigger factor.
E   Aspirin gives relief by reducing the inflammatory reaction.

189 Immunology of allergic rhinitis
A   Most patients have a specific allergy to one substance only.
B   IgE is released by the mast cell.
C   There is a Type I hypersensitivity reaction.
D   Histamine leaks from the endothelial cells via loosened
desmosomal junctions.
E   IgG is involved in some cases.

187

A **F.** The majority can be managed medically. Local steroids have been a great advance.

B **F.** Diathermy to the inferior turbinates, either surface or submucosal, is used to reduce their bulk to help relieve nasal obstruction. Many surgeons believe that pressure of an enlarged middle turbinate on the septum can cause pain, but diathermy is not used for this indication.

C **T.** What appears as a minor deformity can be significant in the context of intermittent mucosal swelling.

D **F.** The operation can cause severe primary or reactionary haemorrhage and should be performed as an in-patient.

E **F.** The long term results are poor, because surgery does not correct the underlying mucosal hyper-reactivity. Vidian neurectomy offers an apparently logical approach to the autonomic imbalance, and is usually effective initially, but in most hands symptoms recur after 2 or 3 years and the operation has lost favour.

188

A **T.**

B **T.** Formed in the nasal mucosa following contact with the allergen, causes release of vasoactive and inflammatory mediators from mast cells.

C **T.**

D **T.** Ingested allergens may also play a role, and there are numerous non-specific additional 'triggers' such as exercise, sudden temperature change, and psychological upset.

E **F.** Aspirin is itself a potent trigger factor, especially in atopic patients with asthma.

189

A **F.** Multiple allergies are the rule, hence the poor success rate of allergen avoidance and desensitization.

B **F.** IgE is released by modified B lymphocytes, plasma cells. It binds to the mast cell causing it to degranulate, releasing histamine, 5-hydroxytryptamine, prostaglandins and leukotrienes, which modulate an acute inflammatory reaction.

C **T.**

D **F.** Histamine is released from mast cells. The tight junctions between the endothelial cells do leak plasma, causing oedema.

E **T.** IgG_4, with a Coombs and Gell Type III reaction.

190 Pathology of allergic rhinitis
A   Oedematous swelling of the mucosa occurs.
B   There is infiltration with giant epithelioid cells.
C   Seromucinous glands atrophy.
D   Venous stasis results in a dusky swelling of the inferior turbinates.
E   Polyp formation is a rare complication.

191 Clinical features of allergic rhinitis
A   Symptoms may be seasonal or perennial.
B   Age of onset is usually in the fourth decade.
C   Anosmia is the main complaint.
D   Sneezing attacks may be incapacitating.
E   Polyps should be suspected if nasal obstruction is permanent.

192 Treatment of allergic rhinitis
A   Avoidance of allergens is frequently impractical.
B   Desensitization based on skin testing is useful in some cases of hay fever.
C   Vasoconstrictor drops provide effective immediate relief.
D   Sedation is the major side effect of antihistamines.
E   Local steroids and sodium cromoglycate both act to reduce the hypersensitivity reaction.

193 Surgical treatment of allergic rhinitis
A   Is preferable to long term medication in children.
B   Is indicated where chronic nasal obstruction is due to polyps.
C   Adenoidectomy is the first line of treatment in children.
D   Reduction of inferior turbinates is indicated for sneezing.
E   Vidian neurectomy can be performed by a transantral approach.

190

A	**T.**	
B	**F.**	Eosinophils and plasma cells predominate. Giant epithelioid cells are a histological feature of tuberculosis.
C	**F.**	They are hyperactive.
D	**T.**	
E	**F.**	Polyps are common.

191

A	**T.**	
B	**F.**	Usually in childhood or early adult life.
C	**F.**	Sneezing, running and blocked nose are the main complaints. Anosmia does occur.
D	**T.**	
E	**T.**	In uncomplicated allergy, the nasal obstruction is intermittent.

192

A	**T.**	Particularly where multiple allergies are present.
B	**T.**	Now carried out much less frequently since the DHSS issued guidelines on the necessity for full cardiopulmonary resuscitation facilities in case of anaphylactic reaction.
C	**T.**	Hence their popularity. The problem is that prolonged use leads to rhinitis medicamentosa.
D	**T.**	This problem has been largely overcome by two modern drugs, terfenadine (Triludan) and astemizole (Hismanal).
E	**T.**	

193

A	**F.**	Surgery is an adjunct rather than an alternative to medical treatment. No operation will cure the underlying allergic tendency.
B	**T.**	
C	**F.**	Allergic rhinitis is not an indication for adenoidectomy.
D	**F.**	Indicated for chronically hypertrophic turbinates causing nasal obstruction. The operation has little or no effect on sneezing or rhinorrhoea.
E	**T.**	

194 Pathology of nasal polyps
A Allergic polyps are usually bilateral.
B Epithelial metaplasia occurs in polyps of vasomotor rhinitis.
C Fibrosis obstructing lymphatic drainage has a role in pathogenesis.
D Malignant polyps are usually indistinguishable from benign clinically.
E Childhood nasal glioma is a malignant polyp.

195 Antrochoanal polyps
A Commonest in the elderly.
B Usually multiple.
C Unilateral nasal obstruction is the commonest symptom.
D The maxillary sinus is opaque on X-rays.
E Most can be completely removed intranasally.

196 Treatment of simple nasal polyps
A Beclomethasone nasal drops will shrink some polyps.
B Systemic steroids are occasionally used in severe cases.
C Antihistamines may improve rhinorrhoea and sneezing.
D Simple snaring of polyps is no longer performed because of the high incidence of recurrence.
E Intranasal ethmoidectomy is the initial treatment of choice.

197 Epiphora
A Is excessive watering of the eye due to nasolacrimal duct or sac obstruction.
B Congenital atresia is the commonest cause.
C May be due to a malignant tumour of the maxillary antrum.
D Initial treatment is by probing the nasolacrimal duct.
E Dacrocystorhinostomy aims to divert tears to the opposite nostril via a plastic tube passed through the septum.

194

A	**T.**	
B	**T.**	A progression from columnar to squamous.
C	**T.**	
D	**F.**	Usually unilateral, may bleed or produce bloody discharge, may cause pain or other local symptoms. Surface appearance varies, may be ulcerated or fleshy, but not typical of benign mucosal variety. Cervical metastases may be present.
E	**F.**	A benign tumour, possibly a hamartoma rather than a true neoplasm.

195

A	**F.**	Adolescents and young adults.
B	**F.**	Single.
C	**T.**	
D	**T.**	
E	**F.**	A Caldwell–Luc approach is often required, although intranasal polypectomy should be tried first. It is helpful when attempting intranasal removal to aspirate fluid via an antral puncture, deflating the antral part of the polyp so that it can be teased out via the ostium.

196

A	**T.**	Up to 50%. Surgery can sometimes be avoided.
B	**T.**	
C	**T.**	
D	**F.**	Although eventual recurrence is common, the procedure is effective and relatively safe. Postoperative local steroid treatment is advised in recurrent cases.
E	**F.**	Overly aggressive for initial treatment. Some surgeons regard intranasal ethmoidectomy as intrinsically dangerous and would go to external ethmoidectomy for severe cases.

197

A	**T.**	
B	**F.**	Chronic dacrocystitis is commonest.
C	**T.**	Sinus X-rays should be performed routinely.
D	**T.**	
E	**F.**	Same side. The sac is opened and sewn to the lateral nasal wall proximal to the site of obstruction.

SECTION 3
THE LARYNX AND TRACHEOBRONCHIAL TREE

198 Development of the larynx
A   The tracheobronchial groove appears cephalic to the hypobranchial eminence.
B   The thyroid cartilage develops from the 4th arch cartilage.
C   The superior laryngeal nerve is the branchial nerve of the 6th arch.
D   The sixth arch artery persists on the left.
E   The early embryonic position of the larynx is high up under the tongue.

199 The infantile larynx in comparison with the adult
A   Is the same relative size.
B   Has its narrowest point in the supraglottis.
C   Lies at a higher level.
D   Collapses easily due to the lack of muscular support.
E   Has an inlet lying less oblique.

200 Cartilaginous framework of the larynx
A   The thyroid alae meet to make an angle of 120° in the female.
B   Calcification of the posterior part of the cricoid lamina can be confused radiographically with a foreign body.
C   The epiglottis is formed of elastic fibrocartilage.
D   The cartilages of Wrisberg do not articulate with any other.
E   The vocal process is completely ossified by 30 years.

201 Laryngeal musculature
A   Only the posterior crico-arytenoid muscle abducts the vocal cords.
B   All the intrinsic muscles are paired.
C   The inferior constrictor steadies the larynx during phonation.
D   Vocalis consists of the lower and deeper fibres of thyro-arytenoid.
E   Contraction of the thyrohyoid can either lower the hyoid or raise the larynx.

198

A	**F.**	It is caudal to it. The tracheobronchial is also called the laryngotracheal groove.
B	**T.**	
C	**F.**	Superior laryngeal nerve supplies the 4th branchial arch; the recurrent laryngeal is the nerve of the 6th arch.
D	**T.**	The ductus arteriosus in the neonate and as the ligamentum arteriosum in the adult. Due to its persistence the left recurrent laryngeal nerve courses through the thorax.
E	**T.**	With maturation it assumes a position lower down, in the adult usually opposite C6/C7.

199

A	**F.**	It is relatively and absolutely smaller.
B	**F.**	Narrowest at the subglottis. Therefore any further constriction by disease rapidly leads to respiratory embarrassment.
C	**T.**	Virtually under the tongue at birth. It descends during growth to lie opposite C6/C7 in the adult.
D	**F.**	Because the laryngeal cartilages are softer than the adult. On forced inspiration they tend to collapse more easily.
E	**T.**	This plane of the laryngeal inlet means a greater risk of aspiration.

200

A	**T.**	In men it is about 90 °. Hence the pronounced 'Adam's apple' in males.
B	**T.**	
C	**T.**	
D	**T.**	Also called cuneiform cartilages. Contained within the mucosa of the aryepiglottic fold.
E	**F.**	It does not ossify.

201

A	**T.**	This paired muscle is the sole abductor.
B	**F.**	All except the transverse arytenoid.
C	**F.**	Although attached to the larynx it has no effect on the vocal function.
D	**T.**	Also called the internal tensor of the vocal cords. The external tensor being the cricothyroid muscle.
E	**T.**	If the hyoid is fixed the larynx is raised and vice versa.

202 In the cavity of the larynx
A   The rima glottidis is the interval between the false cords.
B   Reinke's space lies between the surface epithelium and the deeper elastic layer.
C   Keratinizing stratified squamous epithelium lines the true cords.
D   The posterior part of the ventricular sinus contains the mucus secreting saccule.
E   The paraglottic and pre-epiglottic spaces are continuous.

203 Neurovascular supply and lymphatic drainage of the larynx
A   The main blood supply is from branches of the superior and inferior thyroid arteries.
B   Lymph from the supraglottic larynx drains to the pre-epiglottic and upper deep cervical nodes.
C   The internal branch of the superior laryngeal nerve is entirely motor.
D   The external branch of the superior laryngeal nerve supplies the cricothyroid muscle.
E   The recurrent laryngeal nerve is sensory above the true cords.

204 Examination of the larynx
A   The anterior commissure is easily visualized on indirect laryngoscopy during quiet inspiration.
B   The Negus laryngoscopes have distal illumination.
C   Stroboscopy is of most value in studying vocal cords during quiet respiration.
D   Anteroposterior tomography is valuable in assessing the degree of spread of subglottic carcinoma.
E   A grating sensation on moving the larynx from left to right is abnormal.

202

A **F.** Between the true cords. Has an anterior intermembranous part and a posterior intercartilaginous section.

B **T.** A large potential space in the true cords which may fill with fluid leading to Reinke's oedema.

C **F.** Non-keratinizing.

D **F.** The saccule is located in the anterior part of the sinus. Its secretion constantly lubricates the vocal cords.

E **T.** Important in the spread of tumours.

203

A **T.**

B **T.**

C **F.** Entirely sensory down to the level of the true cords.

D **T.**

E **F.** Sensory below the vocal cords.

204

A **F.** Usually only visualized on vocalization of a high-pitched 'eee'.

B **F.** Negus introduced proximal illumination so as to give an unobstructed lumen. Chevalier Jackson instruments have an electric bulb at the distal end.

C **F.** Stroboscopy gives a slow motion view of the vocal cords during phonation. Particularly useful in the study of speech physiology and in the analysis of abnormal voice production.

D **T.** However, CT scanning is superior as it allows accurate assessment of both soft tissue and skeletal structures.

E **F.** A normal finding as the larynx is separated from the vertebral column only by the thin sheet of prevertebral muscles. This sign may be lost due to carcinoma of the upper aerodigestive tract intervening between laryngeal cartilage and bone.

205 Sphincteric functions of the larynx
A The aryepiglottic sphincter closes during deglutition and vomiting.
B The false cord sphincter is primarily involved in preventing ingress of foreign material.
C The true vocal cords have a curved inferior surface with the concavity directed inferiorly.
D The false cord sphincter cannot be closed independently of the true vocal cords.
E The mechanical mechanism of the true vocal cord sphincter can resist a pharyngeal pressure of 150 mm Hg.

206 During deglutition
A Only the aryepiglottic sphincter closes.
B The larynx is lowered to assist passage of the food bolus into the pharyngo-oesophageal opening.
C Laryngeal airflow continues in an outward direction.
D The epiglottis tilts forwards.
E The lymphocytes in the tonsils sample the food as it passes by.

205

A	**T.**	Its action opposes the aryepiglottic folds. Anteriorly the closure is completed by the epiglottic tubercle and posteriorly by the bodies of the arytenoid cartilages. The epiglottis *per se* is not essential in preventing aspiration as it can be surgically removed without complications.
B	**F.**	It acts as a mechanical flap valve, due to its anatomical shape, preventing egress of air. Hence producing a rise in intratracheal pressure necessary for coughing, sneezing, micturition and parturition. It offers little resistance to the ingress of air but is useful in preventing aspiration of foreign material by physiological muscular contraction.
C	**T.**	This shape offers minimal resistance to air outflow.
D	**T.**	
E	**T.**	Due to the flat upper surface of the true cords, when opposed. The result is a very efficient valve preventing ingress of foreign material.

206

A	**F.**	All three sphincters (aryepiglottic, false cord and true cord) contract reflexly.
B	**F.**	It is elevated to bring about this situation.
C	**F.**	Airflow ceases completely.
D	**F.**	Tilts backwards to help deflect the food into the pyriform fossae.
E	**F.**	A fanciful idea.

207 In voice production
A   The frequency of tone can be altered by adjusting the shape of the free margin of the vocal cords.
B   Articulation is performed by the vibrating cords.
C   Infraglottic air pressure changes do not alter pitch.
D   The neuromuscular theory supposes that vocal cord vibrations are produced by muscle contractions.
E   The aerodynamic theory states that vocal cord vibrations are due to infraglottic pressure.

208 Symptoms and signs of laryngeal disease in the newborn include
A   Failure to thrive.
B   Cough.
C   Tracheal plunging.
D   Croup.
E   Tachycardia.

209 Congenital laryngeal stridor (laryngomalacia)
A   The laryngeal superstructure is soft and may be oedematous.
B   The epiglottis is normal.
C   May present as failure to thrive.
D   Amputation of the epiglottis is effective treatment.
E   The condition usually resolves, without treatment, by age 2 years.

207

A **T.**   Occurs as the voice registers are changed. The edges
are thick in low registers and thin in higher ones. This
alteration is produced by contraction of the deep fibres
of the thyro-arytenoid (vocalis).

B **F.**   The vocal cords phonate, i.e. produce the basic sound
of the voice at a pitch determined by their frequency of
vibration. Timbre is added by the resonating structures
of the vocal tract (pharynx, oral cavity, nose, etc.).
Articulation is the breaking up of the sound into
recognizable language by the coordinated action of the
palate, tongue, jaws and lips.

C **F.**   An increase in infraglottic air pressure leads to a rise in
intensity and a slight increase in pitch.

D **T.**   Although this view is held only by a few. Fibres of the
thyroarytenoid cannot contract at frequencies over
100 Hz without producing tetany. The upper limit of
the human voice being about 2000 Hz.

E **T.**   With contraction of the thyroarytenoid forcing the
cords shut and the infraglottic air pressure forcing
them apart.

208

A **T.**   Breathing and feeding difficulties are usually
associated.

B **T.**   Particularly if there is an irritative lesion in the larynx or
there is overspill into the tracheobronchial tree.

C **T.**   A high negative pressure in the pleural cavity sucks the
larynx and trachea into the thorax.

D **T.**   Croup is the same as inspiratory stridor.

E **T.**   An almost invariable accompaniment of laryngeal
disease.

209

A **T.**

B **F.**   Usually elongated, thin and folded on itself. The so
called 'omega' shape.

C **T.**   Commonest symptom, however, is inspiratory stridor
during sleep.

D **F.**

E **T.**   Although some noise may persist up to 5 years of age.
Rarely, death may occur from chest infections.

210 Congenital laryngeal web

A   Symptoms may be absent.
B   Usually involves the posterior one sixth of the vocal cords.
C   The voice is of normal quality.
D   Excision should be performed as early as possible.
E   The atresia may be a cause of still birth.

211 In closed laryngeal injuries

A   Surgical emphysema can involve the chest and abdomen.
B   The cricoid cartilage is most frequently fractured.
C   A fixed vocal cord is always due to damage to the recurrent laryngeal nerve.
D   Dyspnoea is due to pressure of the cervical vertebrae on the larynx.
E   Perichondritis may be prevented by performing urgent tracheostomy.

210

A	**T.**	If the web is small.
B	**F.**	Anterior one-sixth. The fusion may extend inferiorly to the upper margin of the cricoid cartilage.
C	**F.**	Hoarseness is usually present.
D	**F.**	Most cases do not need treatment. Thin webs can be divided endoscopically, using normal microlaryngeal instruments or laser. Insertion of a keel, either endoscopically or via a laryngofissure approach, will usually be necessary for thicker webs. A tracheostomy may be required for severe stridor or dyspnoea but excision via a laryngofissure should be delayed until the larynx is mature.
E	**T.**	And easily overlooked.

211

A	**T.**	The emphysema starts in the neck and spreads to the face, upper limbs, etc.
B	**F.**	Hyoid and thyroid cartilage fractures are much more common.
C	**F.**	The nerve may be severed. However, haematoma or oedema may compromise its action. Post traumatic fibrosis of the cord or the cricoarytenoid may also fix the cord.
D	**F.**	Due to a submucosal swelling or soft tissue displacement. Mediastinal emphysema will exacerbate the pathology.
E	**F.**	Prevented by administering prophylactic systemic antibiotics and debridement as indicated.

212 Laryngeal trauma

A   If due to an inhalation burn the glottis is oedematous.
B   With an impacted inhaled foreign body Heimlich's manoeuvre
     may be effective in expelling it.
C   The use of relaxant drugs has increased the incidence of
     intubation injuries.
D   Flat foreign bodies in the larynx tend to lie anteroposteriorly in
     the long axis of the larynx.
E   Laryngectomy may be necessary for radiotherapy reaction.

213 Abnormal voice production

A   Violent and forced closure of the vocal cords is a normal
     occurrence during weight lifting.
B   →Tenors are more likely to suffer from vocal nodules than basses.
C   Contact ulcers occur as a result of abnormal approximation of
     the vocal processes of the arytenoid.
D   Mogiphonia is a psychoneurotic form of phonic spasm.
E   Most voice failures in singers are due to inadequate training.

214 Acute non-specific laryngitis in children

A   May be associated with exanthemata
B   May progress to laryngitis stridulosa.
C   Croupy cough is a common symptom.
D   Has to be distinguished from an inhaled foreign body.
E   An oxygen/helium mixture may be beneficial.

212

A **F.** Usually only the supraglottis is involved, the vocal cords being spared.

B **T.** A sudden type of bear hug from behind with the arms encircling the patient just below the xiphisternum. Children can be turned upside down and slapped on the back. Digital extraction via the mouth may be attempted!

C **F.** Reduced them. Intubation injuries are due to traumatic insertion, an oversized tube, an over-inflated cuff, excessive tube movement or prolonged intubation.

D **T.** Therefore may not be seen on AP radiographic views. Flat foreign bodies in the pharynx lie in a transverse plane and may not be seen on a lateral view. Hence, always insist on both views, AP and lateral.

E **T.** Particularly in severe intractable cases with respiratory embarrassment and lack of voice. Also severe reactions may mask the continuing presence or recurrence of tumour.

213

A **T.** Forced expiration against the closed glottis raises intrathoracic pressure to splint the diaphragm. May produce acute submucosal haemorrhage of the vocal cords.

B **T.** Tenors employ the anterior part of the vocal cord for vibrations; the site of vocal nodules. Commoner if the singer employs the 'coup de glotte' or sings outside his / her range, a fault particularly of sopranos.

C **T.** Almost exclusively in adult males who persistently abuse the voice, e.g. street vendors.

D **T.** Occurs particularly in voice professionals such as singers and teachers. The cords go into spasm after uttering a few words in public.

E **T.**

214

A **T.**

B **T.** The name applied when inspiratory stridor is present.

C **T.** It is due to laryngeal spasm.

D **T.** The absence of a raised temperature or other signs of infection should alert the doctor to the possibility of a foreign body.

E **T.** This mixture has a much lower density than air, reducing the resistance to flow through a compromised laryngeal inlet.

215 Acute epiglottitis
A   Inflammatory changes affect mainly the submucosa of the sinus of Morgagni.
B   Pharyngeal symptoms predominate in the adult.
C   Nasotracheal intubation is easily performed.
D   The causal organism is usually a corynebacterium.
E   Systemic steroids are essential.

216 Acute laryngotracheobronchitis
A   Is associated with influenzal epidemics.
B   Produces copious volumes of serous exudate.
C   A relatively quiet chest on auscultation is a good prognostic sign.
D   Must be distinguished from diphtheria.
E   Can lead to rapid overhydration if untreated.

217 Keratosis of the larynx
A   Should be treated with radiotherapy.
B   Produces impairment of cord mobility.
C   Gives a nibbled appearance due to ulceration of the free cord margin.
D   Is characterized by a 'wash-leather' ulceration of the epiglottis.
E   Is a precancerous condition.

215

A	**F.**	Mainly the loosely attached mucosa of the epiglottis.
B	**T.**	In a child laryngeal rather than pharyngeal symptoms are manifest.
C	**F.**	Usually difficult. Also there is a risk of rupturing a supervening epiglottic abscess.
D	**F.**	Invariably *H. influenzae*.
E	**F.**	Although commonly administered their value has never been proven.

216

A	**T.**	It is initiated by a virus, usually Parainfluenza type I. Bacterial infection particularly with *Staphylococcus aureus* may occasionally supervene, causing a very severe form.
B	**F.**	Secretions are thick and tenacious and difficult to expel.
C	**F.**	A quiet or silent chest is a sign of imminent respiratory failure.
D	**T.**	By bacteriological examination. Removal of a diphtheritic membrane causes underlying mucosal bleeding.
E	**F.**	Dehydration is very common and must be actively prevented by intravenous fluid supplements if indicated.

217

A	**F.**	Repeated stripping of the cords is the usual practice unless frank carcinoma supervenes.
B	**F.**	
C	**F.**	This appearance is characteristic of tuberculous laryngitis.
D	**F.**	This appearance is seen in the tertiary form of acquired syphilis and represents the gummatous lesion.
E	**T.**	There is a significant risk of progression to carcinoma *in situ* and frank invasive carcinoma.

218 Juvenile respiratory papillomatosis
   A   Commonly involves the vocal cords and ventricular bands.
   B   Is primarily a disease of young adults.
   C   Should be treated with radiotherapy.
   D   May require laryngectomy.
   E   Is caused by a haemolytic positive streptococcus.

219 Benign lesions of the larynx
   A   Granular cell myoblastoma histologically shows profuse
       pseudo-epitheliomatous hyperplasia.
   B   Retention cysts occur most commonly in the ventricular sinus.
   C   Chondromata usually arise from the arytenoid cartilages.
   D   Benign tumours occur more frequently than malignant tumours.
   E   Adult haemangiomata usually require surgical excision.

218

A	**T.**	May spread to epiglottis, trachea, pharynx and bronchi.
B	**F.**	Infants and young children mostly affected but may continue into adult life. The disease may not involute at puberty.
C	**F.**	This mode of treatment can lead to damage of laryngeal cartilages and there is a risk of malignant change in the long term. Repeated endoscopic removal of the papillomata, with conservation of normal structures, is required. Suction diathermy has recently been superseded by CO_2 laser for this purpose.
D	**T.**	In severe cases of the disease or if stenosis due to scarring occurs. Tracheostomy is sometimes necessary but should be avoided if possible because further spread can occur into the tracheobronchial tree and occasionally into the parenchyma of the lung.
E	**F.**	Caused by the Human Papilloma Virus (HPV) types 6 and 8. HPV type 6 has also been found in genital warts in the mother.

219

A	**T.**	This feature may result in a mistaken diagnosis of squamous cell carcinoma. Malignant change has not been reported.
B	**F.**	Usually on or adjacent to the epiglottis. A potentially fatal condition in young children.
C	**F.**	Uncommon tumour that arises in the subglottis, frequently the posterior plate of the cricoid cartilage.
D	**F.**	Squamous cell carcinoma is the most common.
E	**F.**	These sessile tumours occur in the supraglottis and usually do not cause obstruction or grow. The infantile haemangioma is frequently sited in the subglottis; causes laryngeal obstruction and rarely requires excision or laser therapy.

220 In the 1987 UICC classification of malignant tumours of the larynx

A   The posterior commissure is part of the glottis.

B   A glottic tumour involving both cords with normal mobility and no extension to other sites is a T1b lesion.

C   A tumour limited to the larynx with cord fixation is T3.

D   The presence of 2 cervical lymph node metastases makes the patient Stage IV.

E   A thyroid cartilage chondrosarcoma which has invaded into the thyroid gland is T4.

221 Spread of malignant disease of the larynx

A   Tumours of the anterior commissure can extend directly into the petiolus.

B   The true vocal cords are virtually devoid of lymph vessels.

C   About 40% of tumours of the false cords and ventricular sinuses have metastasized at the time of diagnosis.

D   There is a paucity of transglottic lymph vessels in the vertical plane of the larynx.

E   Epiglottic tumours may metastasize to the submandibular and submental nodes.

220

UICC Classification (1987)

A **T.**   N-staging (all sites)
B **T.**
C **T.**   Ipsilateral single node up to 3 cm N1
D **T.**   Ipsilateral single node 3 to 6 cm N2a
             Ipsilateral multiple nodes up to 6 cm............. N2b
             Bilateral/contralateral nodes up to 6 cm........ N2c
             Any node greater than 6 cm........................ N3

Stage grouping

Stage	T	N	M
Stage 0	Tis	N0	M0
Stage I	T1	N0	M0
Stage II	T2	N0	M0
Stage III	T3	N0	M0
	T1–3	N1	M0
Stage IV	T4	N0,1	M0
	T any	N2,3	M0
	T any	N any	M1

E **F.**   The classification only applies to squamous carcinoma.

221

A **T.**   Usually at an early stage. Can also invade the thyroid cartilage. This site carries a poor prognosis.
B **T.**   Hence the more favourable prognosis and the basis of limited local excision such as cordectomy.
C **T.**   Because of the abundant lymphatics which crossflow making contralateral and bilateral nodal pathology very likely.
D **T.**   This is the pathophysiological basis of a partial supraglottic laryngectomy. Transglottic tumours are likely to be due to direct growth in both directions spread.
E **T.**   More commonly the upper and middle deep cervical nodes. Bilateral nodal disease from this midline structure is not uncommon.

222 Total laryngectomy

A   Billroth of Vienna was the first to perform the procedure for cancer of the larynx.
B   The Sorenson U flap incision may be unsatisfactory after high dose radiotherapy.
C   The inferior constrictor is the most important structure in the repair of the pharyngeal wall.
D   Postoperatively a laryngectomy tube is essential for a few days.
E   Prophylactic use of metronidazole has reduced the incidence of postoperative pharyngocutaneous fistula.

223 Laryngocoeles

A   Are caused by dilatation of the subglottis.
B   The external variety project through the thyrohyoid membrane.
C   Can easily be demonstrated with plain X-rays.
D   Early excision is advisable.
E   May be caused by tumour.

224 Oedema of the larynx

A   The glottis is the site most frequently affected.
B   An idiosyncrasy to iodine may be an aetiological factor.
C   A mixture of oxygen and helium may be useful.
D   0.5 ml of 1 : 1000 adrenaline should be given intramuscularly in an adult.
E   Stertorous breathing implies supraglottic pathology.

222

A **T.**   In 1874. However, a Scot, Patrick Heron Watson performed the first ever total laryngectomy for syphilis in 1866.

B **T.**   The tip may necrose. But is frequently employed as it has the advantages of good exposure, easier suturing around the tracheostome and skin incisions are distant from the pharyngeal repair sutures.

C **T.**   The pharyngeal defect should be sutured in two layers. The first being a continuous extramucosal inverting suture layer which includes the constrictor. The second interrupted layer is a reinforcement and should cover the first suture lines. The stitch pattern should be a horizontal line as this appears to increase the chances of acquiring oesophageal speech and use an artificial valve apparatus.

D **F.**   If the skin to tracheal mucosa suture is precise no tube is required.

E **T.**

223

A **F.**   Dilatation of the ventricular saccule of the larynx. They are usually bilateral.

B **T.**   The internal laryngocoele resembles a cyst underneath the ventricular band.

C **T.**   Particularly during forced Valsalva manoeuvre.

D **F.**   Only if symptoms of hoarseness or dyspnoea are troublesome. The internal laryngocoele can be uncapped endoscopically and the external variety by an external approach that may include division of the thyroid cartilage.

E **T.**   Neoplasia should be excluded in all cases.

224

A **F.**   Occurs in areas where the mucosa is loosely adherent. Namely the supraglottis (vestibule and aryepiglottic folds) in adults and subglottis in children. The epiglottis may become oedematous secondary to infection and is potentially lethal in children.

B **T.**   An allergic phenomenon producing rapid anaphylaxis (Angioneurotic oedema). Aspirin and certain food substances are also potential allergens.

C **T.**   This mixture facilitates the flow of oxygen through the obstructive area.

D **F.**   Given subcutaneously. In a child an initial dose of 0.1 ml is sufficient.

E **T.**   Muffled and high pitched respiration is more likely with problems of the glottis and subglottis.

225 In episodes of stridor
A   Laryngismus stridulus is accompanied by a pyrexia.
B   An inhaled foreign body should be excluded.
C   A vocal cord paralysis may be present.
D   If due to laryngomalacia the prognosis is good.
E   In an infant with a normal appearance of the larynx an enlarged thymus may exist.

226 Neural paralysis of the larynx
A   Aspiration is more likely if the superior laryngeal nerve is affected.
B   The paralysed cord usually lies at a lower level.
C   If due to bronchial carcinoma the primary pathology is easily diagnosed in most cases.
D   Semon's law states that in a progressive lesion the adductors are affected before the abductors.
E   The cartilage of Wrisberg becomes more prominent.

227 Management of laryngeal paralysis
A   A unilateral recurrent laryngeal nerve paralysis may recover.
B   If due to mediastinal spread from carcinoma of the oesophagus indicates a possibility of surgical cure.
C   Laser arytenoidectomy is useful in unilateral lesions.
D   Cordopexy obviates the need for a tracheostomy in bilateral recurrent nerve lesions.
E   Teflon paste injection for unilateral paralysis is of little value.

228 Voice disorders
A   Due to myotonia atrophica may produce phonaesthenia.
B   Of functional origin usually have an abnormal cough.
C   Due to closure of the false cords are commonly psychogenic.
D   Such as dysphonia plicae ventricularis may be caused by compensatory efforts in vocal disabilities.
E   Due to ventricular band movements are best treated with speech therapy.

225

A	**F.**	Usually apyrexial. Most common in young boys and may be associated with carpo pedal spasm.
B	**T.**	
C	**T.**	Both unilateral and bilateral recurrent laryngeal nerve palsies may produce dyspnoea/stridor only during an upper respiratory tract infection.
D	**T.**	Most children will improve spontaneously with age.
E	**T.**	

226

A	**T.**	There is loss of sensation in the supraglottis.
B	**T.**	
C	**T.**	Usually obvious on the chest X-ray. However in rare cases a left recurrent nerve paralysis may appear before there is any evidence of lung carcinoma.
D	**F.**	The reverse is true. The phylogenetically older adductors are not as vulnerable as the more recent abductors.
E	**T.**	Particularly in lesions of the recurrent nerve.

227

A	**T.**	Particularly if idiopathic in origin. After thyroidectomy the nerve may recover if it was noted to be intact during the procedure.
B	**F.**	Indicates inoperability. The same is true of bronchial carcinoma.
C	**F.**	May be employed in bilateral recurrent nerve palsies.
D	**T.**	This is its only advantage. The voice is often imperfect.
E	**F.**	A very valuable procedure. In idiopathic cases it should be employed only after a lapse of 9 months and after intensive speech therapy. It is the treatment of choice for recurrent nerve lesions due to carcinoma of the lung, oesophagus and breast.

228

A	**T.**	A rare cause of phonaesthenia. Other aetiological factors leading to this condition include myasthenia gravis, laryngeal TB, vocal misuse, laryngitis and extreme weight loss.
B	**F.**	The cough is nearly always normal and the cords are seen to adduct fully.
C	**T.**	
D	**T.**	Particularly compensation in myasthenia. False cord opposition produces an extremely rough voice.
E	**T.**	

229 Development of the trachea and bronchi
A   The laryngotracheal groove appears at about 25 weeks of embryonic life.
B   Approximately 20 million alveoli are present at birth.
C   The lung bud forms 3 lobules on the left side.
D   The non-respiratory bronchiolar division is complete by birth.
E   The number of alveoli does not increase after birth.

230 In the trachea
A   The carina has an external landmark at the level of the sternal angle.
B   A 'forceps space' occurs around a foreign body.
C   The mucosal lining is transitional ciliated columnar epithelium.
D   The first and second tracheal rings are not infrequently fused.
E   The recurrent laryngeal nerve supplies the trachea.

231 In the neck
A   The recurrent nerves lie in the groove between trachea and vertebral bodies.
B   The thymus lies behind the trachea.
C   The thyroid isthmus is at a higher level in children than adults.
D   Lymphatic drainage is to the deep cervical nodes.
E   The recurrent nerves always pass in front of the inferior thyroid artery.

232 In the tracheobronchial tree
A   A bronchopulmonary segment consists of a segment of lung with its segmental bronchus.
B   Aspiration in a supine patient is most likely to cause problems in the apical bronchus of the right lower lobe.
C   The left brachiocephalic vein is anterior to the thoracic trachea.
D   Respiratory bronchioles are supported by complete rings of cartilage.
E   The carina is 25 cm from the incisor teeth in an adult.

229

A **T.** Also called the tracheobronchial groove. Located in the primitive pharynx.

B **T.** Which by age 8 have reached the adult number of about 300 million.

C **F.** Three on the right and two on the left.

D **T.**

E **F.** It is the propagation of alveoli that increases the lung size (see B above).

230

A **T.** The second costal cartilage. The precise position is dependent on posture and the respiratory cycle.

B **T.** The bronchial diameter increases during inspiration and allows easier passage of forceps for removal of a foreign body.

C **F.** Pseudostratified ciliated columnar epithelium with an abundance of goblet cells.

D **T.**

E **T.** The recurrent nerve is both motor and sensory to the trachea.

231

A **F.** In the groove between trachea and oesophagus.

B **F.** Anterior to it at the root of the neck. Present only in children.

C **T.** In adults it usually crosses the 2, 3 and 4th tracheal rings.

D **F.** To the pre- and paratracheal nodes.

E **F.** Can be in front, behind or amongst the terminal branches of the inferior thyroid artery.

232

A **T.**

B **T.** A frequent site of pneumonitis, collapse or abscess formation.

C **T.** But may project superiorly and hence be in danger during tracheostomy. In infants the brachiocephalic artery may produce similar complications because of its higher position.

D **F.** Cartilage support in the tracheobronchial system occurs only as far as bronchioles of 1 mm diameter.

E **T.** A useful landmark when an orotracheal tube is inserted.

233 In the upper air passages
A   The length of cervical trachea can alter in any one individual.
B   The trachea is nearest to the skin at the 4th tracheal ring.
C   The larynx descends during postnatal growth.
D   The pleural dome is at risk during tracheostomy.
E   The cricoid cartilage may be more easily palpated than the thyroid cartilage.

234 In performing a tracheostomy
A   The head should be extended to a maximum degree.
B   A vertical tracheal incision should be avoided in children.
C   The tracheal incision should always include the first tracheal ring.
D   The tracheostomy tube should fit tightly without a cuff.
E   Tapes should be tied with the head in the neutral position.

235 In the postoperative care of tracheostomy
A   A postoperative lateral cervical X-ray should be performed.
B   Accidental decannulation after 2 weeks should be treated as an emergency.
C   Copious mucus production indicates a pulmonary infection.
D   A poorly positioned tracheostomy tube may produce a fatal haemorrhage.
E   Mucus and crusts are the commonest causes of obstruction.

233

A	**T.**	It varies with physique and degree of neck extension.
B	**F.**	Immediately below the cricoid cartilage.
C	**T.**	From C3 in the infant to about C6 in the adult.
D	**T.**	Contents of the mediastinum may enter the neck when the latter is extended. In particular the pleural domes and left brachiocephalic vein. In infants the thymus and brachiocephalic artery.
E	**T.**	Particularly in infants as the definitive configuration of the thyroid cartilage takes place at puberty.

234

A	**F.**	Such a manoeuvre may lead to both skin incision and tracheal fenestration being placed too low. In an adult postoperative nursing may be difficult and in a neonate the stoma may end up behind the manubrium. Additionally there is the risk of drawing up mediastinal contents into the neck during the procedure (e.g. brachiocephalic vessels).
B	**F.**	It is the most suitable incision, giving the least risk of transection and in the long term results in less stenosis and airways resistance. A Bjork flap should be avoided as there is a risk of detachment into the tracheal lumen.
C	**F.**	It predisposes to subglottic stenosis.
D	**T.**	Should be a loose fit. A high volume low pressure cuff should be employed to reduce the risk of ischaemic damage to the mucosa with subsequent ulceration, granulation, and cartilage necrosis with stenosis.
E	**F.**	The head should be slightly flexed.

235

A	**T.**	Both lateral and PA views to ensure that the tracheostomy tube is not sited in the anterior tracheal space. In children, a tube that is too long, and lodged in the right main bronchus, can be demonstrated.
B	**F.**	The fistula tract should be mature but the matter requires urgent attention.
C	**F.**	The tracheobronchial secretions increase in volume and is a normal reaction. It does not indicate infection but this may supervene if regular suction is not performed or the mucus dries and a crust obstructs the lung causing atelectasis.
D	**T.**	A tracheostomy tube tip may erode the anterior tracheal wall and the brachiocephalic artery.
E	**T.**	Others include a prolapsed cuff or an infant's chin.

236 In a child with a tracheostomy
A   Endoscopy prior to decannulation is useful rather than essential in long standing cases.
B   There may be a predisposition to recurrent chest infections.
C   A suprastomal granulation may result in decannulation difficulties.
D   Surgical decannulation may result in surgical emphysema.
E   The mortality of the procedure is about 1%.

237 Congenital abnormalities of the tracheobronchial tree
A   Account for less than 10% of cases of congenital stridor.
B   Include bulging of the posterior tracheal wall.
C   Producing tracheomalacia are most commonly due to internal compression.
D   Resulting in posterior tracheal compression occurs with an aberrant left subclavian artery.
E   Vascular compression of the trachea with severe symptoms is best managed by tracheostomy.

238 The following are indications necessitating tracheostomy
A   A child with acute laryngotracheobronchitis.
B   Patients in whom endotracheal intubation is continued for more than about 3 weeks.
C   A single failed attempt at endotracheal intubation in a child with acute supraglottitis.
D   Total maxillectomy.
E   Laryngeal trauma with evidence of frothy blood.

236

A **F.** Essential. It allows assessment of the suprastomal region for granulations, subglottic narrowing, tracheal wall collapse and vocal cord movements.

B **T.** The child may benefit from a trial of decannulation.

C **T.** It causes tracheal narrowing above the stoma. Additional problems are due to a flap of fibrous tissue or a displaced anterior tracheal wall in the same region.

D **T.** Particularly if the tracheal stoma is inadequately sutured.

E **F.** About 5%. However endotracheal intubation has largely superseded it for many inflammatory pathologies.

237

A **F.** About 25%.

B **F.** A normal finding in neonates due to laxity of the trachealis.

C **F.** The localized form is due to external compression. The less common generalized form usually recovers spontaneously although occasionally requires insertion of a long length tracheostomy tube.

D **F.** Aberrant right subclavian artery passes between trachea and oesophagus and produces symptoms referable to one or both structures. An aberrant left subclavian artery compresses the oesophagus alone as it passes posterior to it.

E **F.** Tracheostomy should be avoided due to the risk of erosion of the artery by the tube tip. Patients with significant symptoms should have a surgical decompression via thoracotomy.

238

A **F.** Only about 1% of these cases require tracheostomy. If an alternative airway is required, the treatment of choice is endotracheal intubation, provided experienced nursing staff are available.

B **T.** Even if low pressure cuffs are employed.

C **T.** Further attempts at endotracheal intubation merely increase soft tissue oedema. A rigid bronchoscope can usually be inserted behind the epiglottis into the trachea and a tracheostomy performed.

D **F.**

E **T.** Most moderate to severe laryngeal trauma cases require an alternative airway. Frothy blood indicates both laryngeal disruption and severe haemorrhage.

239 Tracheobronchial foreign bodies
A   Are most common between ages 10 and 15 years.
B   May cause an initial episode of choking.
C   May present as a unilateral wheeze.
D   Can cause a haemoptysis.
E   Become symptomatic within a few days.

240 In the management of an inhaled foreign body
A   The chest X-ray is always abnormal if the site of impaction is the bronchus.
B   Conservative management should be employed initially.
C   A combined bronchoscope and grasping forceps is useful for soft vegetable foreign bodies.
D   The Clerf–Arrowsmith forceps are useful for removing peanuts.
E   Steroids should always be administered post removal.

241 Inflammatory processes in the tracheobronchial tree
A   Tracheitis sicca may be improved by laryngectomy.
B   Dextrocardia may rarely be present.
C   Acute laryngotracheobronchitis is more common in boys.
D   Antitoxins are not required if tracheal diphtheria is treated with systemic penicillin.
E   Foreign bodies should always be excluded.

239

A	**F.**	76% of inhaled foreign bodies occur in children below 4 years of age.
B	**T.**	Usually preceded by paroxysmal coughing.
C	**T.**	In a child without asthma this symptom should lead to a search for an inhaled foreign body.
D	**T.**	Particularly if vegetable in type as it causes a florid mucosal reaction with marked granulations.
E	**F.**	After the initial choking, etc., symptoms may cease. This may be the case for several months if the foreign body is made of an inert substance producing little mucosal irritation.

240

A	**F.**	The chest X-ray may be entirely normal. However, classical changes can occur if there is obstruction of the smaller airways. Namely, over inflation of the lung, atelectasis and pneumonic changes. The foreign body may also be radio-opaque. Mediastinal emphysema may be seen if the airway has been punctured by a sharp object.
B	**F.**	The value of bronchodilators, postural drainage and thoracic percussion is limited. There is a danger of the foreign body impacting in the subglottis. Rigid endoscopy is mandatory.
C	**T.**	The large jaws prevent fragmentation.
D	**F.**	For removal of safety pins.
E	**F.**	Not usually necessary. Indicated if the procedure is prolonged or there is a risk of subglottic oedema, particularly in children.

241

A	**F.**	May be caused by it. Occasionally associated with atrophic rhinitis and laryngitis sicca. The dry crusts require humidification to soften them and occasionally formal toilet to remove them.
B	**T.**	Kartagener's, syndrome i.e. bronchiectasis, chronic sinusitis and dextrocardia.
C	**T.**	Usually under 4 years of age. Caused most frequently by para-influenza virus type 1.
D	**F.**	Antitoxins are essential to neutralize the exotoxins that can produce myocarditis and peripheral neuritis.
E	**T.**	Particularly in children and in those with recurrent problems or unilateral signs.

242 In carcinoma of the bronchus
A   A persistent unproductive cough is an early symptom.
B   Only hilar invasion causes hoarseness by involvement of the left recurrent laryngeal nerve.
C   Ptosis may be associated with paralysis of the hand.
D   Dysphonia caused by cord palsy should be treated with a course of speech therapy.
E   Presentation may be with an enlarging cervical node.

243 Management of benign tracheal stenosis
A   Tracheomalacia is often misdiagnosed as stenosis.
B   Up to 8 cm of trachea can be excised and an end to end anastamosis still possible.
C   Laser excision has replaced repeat dilatations.
D   Grillo and Barclay described the same procedure.
E   Marlex mesh is of great value in strengthening the tracheal wall.

242

   A   **T.**   Later to become productive of purulent and bloodstained sputum.

   B   **F.**   Apical tumour may compromise either recurrent nerve and cause similar symptoms.

   C   **T.**   By an apical tumour (Pancoast's) invading the brachial plexus (shoulder pain and hand paralysis) and the cervical sympathetic chain (Horner's syndrome— ptosis, meiosis, enophthalmos and loss of facial sweating).

   D   **F.**   The patient is incurable and requires immediate surgical management by Teflon paste injection. This improves amplitude, prevents aspiration and enhances expectoration.

   E   **T.**   Lymphatic spread is usually to the hilar nodes but can occur in the supraclavicular nodes.

243

   A   **T.**   With tracheomalacia both endoscopy and X-ray will reveal a normal trachea.

   B   **F.**   An upper limit of 5 cm only. The mediastinal trachea has to be mobilized and a laryngeal drop performed.

   C   **F.**   Both are useful procedures. Very minor degrees of stenosis are probably best treated with dilatations.

   D   **T.**   Grillo (USA) and Barclay (UK). Involves resection of the stenotic segment and primary anastamosis of the stumps after resiting the right main bronchus into the left main bronchus.

   E   **F.**   Very rarely successful. It frequently migrates and is a nidus for infection.

SECTION 4
MOUTH, PHARYNX AND OESOPHAGUS

244 Development of the mouth
A   The stomatodeum or primitive mouth lies between the frontonasal process cranially and first branchial arch caudally.
B   The stomatodeum is lined by ectoderm.
C   The buccopharyngeal membrane separates the stomatodeum from the primitive pharynx.
D   The primitive pharynx is lined by endoderm.
E   Rathke's pouch is an ectodermal derivative.

245 Development of the tongue
A   The anterior two thirds develop from the second branchial arch.
B   The posterior one third develops from the copula.
C   Internal musculature is derived from suboccipital myotomes.
D   The foramen caecum is the lingual opening of the thyroglossal duct.
E   The glossopharyngeal nerve supplies third arch structures.

246 Development of the pharynx
A   The supratonsillar fossa is a derivative of the second pharyngeal pouch.
B   The glossopharyngeal nerve supplies second pouch derivatives.
C   Tonsillar lymphatic tissue is of mesodermal origin.
D   The cervical sinus (of His) normally communicates with the lumen of the pharynx.
E   The hypopharynx is derived from the fifth pharyngeal pouch.

244

A	**T.**	
B	**T.**	
C	**T.**	Breaks down early, approx. 4 weeks.
D	**T.**	As is the remainder of the GI tract.
E	**T.**	Forms the anterior pituitary.

245

A	**F.**	The anterior two thirds is formed from the fusion of two lateral tubercles and the tuberculum impar. All are first arch derivatives.
B	**T.**	A midline derivative of the third arch, also known as the hypobranchial eminence.
C	**T.**	Supplied by the hypoglossal nerve.
D	**T.**	
E	**T.**	

246

A	**T.**	From its ventral diverticulum. The dorsal diverticulum forms part of the tubotympanic recess.
B	**T.**	The facial nerve is also involved.
C	**T.**	All lymphatic tissue is of mesodermal origin.
D	**F.**	The cervical sinus is formed by a ventral overgrowth of the second arch, which comes to overlie the remaining arches and clefts caudal to it. It fuses with the neck skin (C2) burying the ectoderm of the third, fourth and sixth arches. There is normally no communication through endodermal lining with the lumen of the pharynx. However, in some cases of branchial fistula, the endoderm does break down. It is usually the second pouch which does so, therefore the internal opening of the fistula is above the tonsil.
E	**F.**	The fifth pouch disappears early, though it may form the ultimobranchial body, which may form the calcitonin secreting C cells of the thyroid.

247 The second pharyngeal pouch
A   Is lined by ectoderm.
B   Has dorsal and ventral diverticula.
C   Forms the eustachian tube.
D   Contributes to the formation of the middle ear.
E   Forms the supratonsillar fossa.

248 Anatomy of the mouth
A   The vestibule is that part of the oral cavity in front of molar teeth.
B   The posterior limit of the oral cavity is the posterior faucial pillar (palatopharyngeal fold).
C   The mouth is lined by stratified squamous epithelium.
D   The parotid duct of Stensen opens opposite the lower second molar tooth.
E   Mandibular and maxillary divisions of the trigeminal nerve supply the mouth.

249 Dental anatomy
A   The deciduous teeth consist of two incisors, one canine and two molars in each half jaw.
B   There are 32 permanent teeth.
C   Teeth develop from ectoderm only.
D   The teeth of the upper jaw are supplied via the anterior, middle and posterior superior alveolar nerves.
E   The apex of the root of the lower third molar lies below the mylohyoid line.

250 Anatomy of the nasopharynx
A   The lower boundary of the nasopharynx is the anterior faucial pillar.
B   The eustachian tube opens at the level of the inferior turbinate.
C   Squamous epithelium lines the normal nasopharynx.
D   Passavant's muscle is made up of fibres of palatopharyngeus.
E   The internal carotid artery is in close relation to the lateral nasopharyngeal recess (Fossa of Rosenmuller).

247

A	**F.**	All the pharyngeal pouches are lined by endoderm.
B	**T.**	
C	**F.**	The eustachian tube is derived from the first pouch (tubotympanic recess) with a contribution from the otic capsule.
D	**T.**	The dorsal diverticulum becomes part of the tubotympanic recess. It carries a pretrematic nerve, the tympanic branch of the glossopharyngeal, into the middle ear.
E	**T.**	

248

A	**F.**	The vestibule is the space between the teeth and gums and the lips and cheeks. It opens into the oral cavity between the teeth and behind the last molars.
B	**F.**	The anterior faucial pillar marks the boundary between mouth and oropharynx.
C	**T.**	
D	**F.**	Opposite the upper second molar tooth.
E	**T.**	The greater and lesser palatine nerves are from the maxillary division, the lingual from the mandibular.

249

A	**T.**	
B	**T.**	Two incisors, one canine, two premolar and three molar in each half jaw.
C	**F.**	The enamel is ectodermal, but the dentine and cementum are mesodermal.
D	**T.**	
E	**T.**	The clinical significance of this is that an apical abscess may point in the neck.

250

A	**F.**	The lower boundary of the nasopharynx is the soft palate. The anterior faucial pillar demarcates mouth from oropharynx.
B	**T.**	
C	**F.**	Pseudostratified ciliated columnar (respiratory) epithelium.
D	**T.**	The lateral fibres pass inside superior constrictor and join posteriorly to form the velopharyngeal sphincter.
E	**T.**	This was a hazard of eustachian tube catheterization, a procedure that is seldom performed since the advent of ventilation tubes (grommets).

251 Anatomy of the oropharynx
A   The upper border of the oropharynx is at the level of the soft palate.
B   The posterior third of the tongue is part of the oropharynx.
C   The posterior boundary of the vallecula is the epiglottis.
D   The oropharynx is lined by squamous epithelium.
E   The palatine tonsil lies between the palatopharyngeal fold anteriorly and the palatoglossal fold posteriorly.

252 The pharyngeal constrictor muscles
A   The pharyngobasilar fascia lies outside the constrictors.
B   Superior constrictor forms part of the tonsillar fossa.
C   Middle constrictor has attachments to the hyoid bone and stylohyoid ligament.
D   Killian's dehiscence is the gap between middle and inferior constrictors.
E   The motor nerve supply is from the pharyngeal plexus via accessory and vagus nerves, with cell bodies in the nucleus ambiguus.

251

A   **T.**   The oropharynx extends from the junction of hard and soft palate to the floor of the vallecula at the level of the hyoid bone. It is bounded anteriorly by the palatoglossal fold which demarcates it from the mouth. There is disagreement between the UICC (International Union Against Cancer) and AJC (American Joint Committee) on the status of the anterior surface of the epiglottis; the UICC places it in the oropharynx while the AJC regards this site as part of the larynx.

B   **T.**

C   **T.**

D   **T.**   Non-keratinizing stratified squamous epithelium.

E   **F.**   The palatopharyngeal fold is posterior and the palatoglossal anterior.

252

A   **F.**   It lies inside.

B   **T.**   The fibres are seen during tonsillectomy, running obliquely across the fossa. They can be divided to gain access to the glossopharyngeal nerve in cases of glossopharyngeal neuralgia. An elongated styloid process is approached in the same way in the treatment of Eagle's syndrome.

C   **T.**   It originates in the acute angle formed by the stylohyoid ligament and the greater cornu of the hyoid.

D   **F.**   Killian's dehiscence is the potential gap which occurs posteriorly between the two parts of inferior constrictor, thyropharyngeus and cricopharyngeus. It is a weak point and is the usual site of origin of a pharyngeal pouch (Zenker's diverticulum).

E   **T.**

253 Anatomy of the palatine tonsil
A   The crypts are lined by squamous epithelium.
B   There are no afferent lymphatics.
C   The tonsillar artery is a branch of the greater palatine.
D   Pain sensation from the tonsil is carried in the glossopharyngeal nerve.
E   The size of the tonsil can be assessed accurately by looking in the mouth while using a tongue depressor.

254 The parapharyngeal space
A   Has no anatomical floor, allowing communication from skull base to superior mediastinum.
B   There is free communication with the retropharyngeal space.
C   The deep lobe of the parotid projects into its lateral wall.
D   Contents include the carotid sheath, the lower four cranial nerves, and deep cervical lymph nodes.
E   At the level of C5 vertebra, the lateral wall is formed by the sternomastoid muscle.

253

A **T.**   Non-keratinizing stratified squamous epithelium covers the pharyngeal surface and extends into all the crypts. Desquamated cells form part of the crypt debris which can be seen as white or yellow spots.

B **T.**   The tonsil acts as an initial antigen processing station for swallowed material, some of which is trapped in the crypts. Efferent lymphatics drain to the jugulo-digastric node.

C **F.**   The tonsillar artery is a branch of the facial. There are some minor branches from the greater palatine which may supply the upper pole. Further blood supply is obtained from small branches of the lingual and ascending pharyngeal arteries.

D **T.**   Hence pain may be referred to the ear.

E **F.**   Some tonsils appear large because the tonsillar fossae are shallow, while others of similar or greater mass may be almost completely buried. In addition, contraction of the pharyngeal musculature can bring the tonsils closer to the midline, so the apparent size is variable in the individual patient. Tonsils which appear large are best described as 'prominent'.

254

A **T.**   Therefore infections can spread intracranially and into the mediastinum. Conversely, middle ear infection can spread via involvement of the jugular foramen or petrous apex into the neck.

B **F.**   There is a condensation of fascia around the carotid sheath which separates parapharyngeal and retropharyngeal spaces. Bilateral spread of infection in the neck is rare.

C **T.**   A deep lobe parotid tumour is a common cause of a mass in the parapharyngeal space. They are usually situated anterior to the styloid process, whereas vascular and neurogenous tumours occur posteriorly—a helpful point in differential diagnosis by CT or MRI scanning.

D **T.**   Other contents are the ascending pharyngeal and palatine arteries, the sympathetic chain and the styloid group of muscles.

E **T.**   In drainage of a parapharyngeal abscess the approach is anterior to sternomastoid for an abscess low in the neck and posterior to the muscle for an abscess high in the neck.

255 The retropharyngeal space

A   Is bounded posteriorly by the prevertebral fascia, anteriorly by the buccopharyngeal fascia, and laterally by the carotid sheath.

B   Extends from skull base to superior mediastinum.

C   Contains the vertebral arteries.

D   Contains the cervical nerve roots.

E   A retropharyngeal abscess usually points in the anterior triangle of the neck.

256 The glossopharyngeal nerve

A   Roots emerge from the midbrain.

B   Exits the skull via the anterior compartment of the jugular foramen.

C   Supplies taste and common sensation to the posterior two thirds of the tongue.

D   Parasympathetic cell bodies for supply of the submandibular gland lie in the superior (petrous) ganglion.

E   The tympanic branch (Jacobson's nerve) contains both sensory and parasympathetic secretomotor fibres.

257 Lymphatic drainage of the pharynx

A   All areas of the pharynx drain ultimately to the lower deep cervical group of nodes.

B   The nasopharynx drains via retropharyngeal and upper deep cervical nodes.

C   The tonsil drains to the jugulodigastric node.

D   The base of the tongue has very little lymphatic drainage.

E   The pyriform fossa may drain to paratracheal nodes.

255

A **T.**

B **T.**

C **F.** The space contains only loose areolar tissue and the retropharyngeal lymph nodes of Rouvier.

D **F.**

E **F.** The abscess may point into the pharynx, as a swelling on the posterior pharyngeal wall, or into the posterior triangle of the neck. An acute abscess is commoner in infants and results from suppuration in the retropharyngeal lymph nodes following an upper respiratory tract infection. It is best drained through the mouth. A chronic abscess occurs in adults due to tuberculosis. The cervical vertebrae may be involved. If drainage is required an external approach through the neck is necessary.

256

A **F.** Roots emerge from the hindbrain, between olive and inferior cerebellar peduncle.

B **T.** A fibrous septum of dura separates the glossopharyngeal nerve and inferior petrosal sinus from the vagus and accessory nerves. However in clinical practice a jugular foramen lesion will usually affect all three nerves.

C **F.** Posterior one third of the tongue, together with tonsils, soft palate, and middle ear. These are third arch and second pouch structures.

D **F.** Parasympathetic cell bodies of the glossopharyngeal nerve are in the otic ganglion, and they supply the parotid. The submandibular gland is supplied from the nervus intermedius via the chorda tympani. The cell bodies in the petrous ganglion of the glossopharyngeal are sensory.

E **T.**

257

A **T.**

B **T.**

C **T.**

D **F.** There is rich bilateral drainage, hence the high incidence of neck metastases in carcinoma of the tongue base.

E **T.**

258 Immunology of the pharyngeal lymphoid tissue
A   B lymphocytes proliferate in active follicles.
B   T lymphocytes secrete lymphokines which act locally to control the inflammatory response.
C   B lymphocytes synthesize IgA secretory antibodies.
D   Macrophages are involved in presenting antigen to T lymphocytes.
E   T lymphocytes are required for cell-mediated immunity.

259 Anatomy of the parotid gland
A   Develops as an ectodermal diverticulum of the primitive oral cavity.
B   Is covered on its outer aspect by a thickened layer of deep cervical fascia.
C   Occupies the space between the mastoid process posteriorly and the ascending ramus of the mandible anteriorly.
D   The facial nerve trunk is deep to the retromandibular vein.
E   Secretomotor fibres to the gland travel in the auriculotemporal nerve.

258

A **T.**   The follicles are similar to those found in lymph nodes, but in the pharyngeal lymphoid tissue there are no afferent lymphatics.

B **T.**   Lymphokines include Migration Inhibition Factor (MIF) which localizes macrophages and monocytes at the inflammatory site, Macrophage Activating Factor (MAF), Interleukin 2 which amplifies the response of antigen-reactive T cells, and the interferons which block transmission of virus particles between cells.

C **T.**   Some of these B cells transform into plasma cells. The secretory IgA is joined into a dimeric form with a secretory protein by epithelial cells. It is then released onto the lumenal surface of the mucosa. There it has neutralizing activity against viruses and toxins, and is able to inhibit many microorganisms from adhering to the epithelial surface.

D **T.**

E **T.**   The T cell is central in control of the entire immune response, but is particularly critical in dealing with microorganisms which are able to 'take up residence' inside the cell. These include viruses, mycobacteria and protozoa. Cell mediated immunity is also required to eliminate fungal infections.

259

A **T.**   This is initially a solid cord, it subsequently arborizes and canalizes.

B **T.**   The thick, unyielding parotid fascia accounts for the severe pain of parotitis. It may also prevent a parotid swelling from becoming obvious until it has reached a large size.

C **T.**

D **F.**   The nerve is superficial to the vein. The external carotid artery is deeper still.

E **T.**   Following parotidectomy, these fibres may reinnervate sweat glands in the skin, leading to Frey's syndrome of gustatory sweating.

260 Anatomy of the submandibular gland
A   The superficial lobe is larger than the deep lobe.
B   Hyoglossus muscle divides deep from superficial lobe.
C   The duct opens laterally in the floor of the mouth opposite the second molar tooth.
D   The mandibular division of the facial nerve lies superficial to the capsule of the gland.
E   The facial artery crosses the gland.

261 The infratemporal fossa
A   Lies below the posterior cranial fossa.
B   Has no anatomical floor.
C   Posterior boundary is the styloid apparatus and carotid sheath.
D   The maxillary artery and maxillary nerve pass through it.
E   Contains the pterygoid venous plexus.

262 The temporomandibular joint
A   Is a synovial joint.
B   Allows both gliding and hinge movements.
C   The medial pterygoid muscle inserts into the articular disc.
D   Jaw opening is initiated by contraction of the lateral pterygoid muscle.
E   Nerve supply is from the maxillary division of the trigeminal.

260

A	**T.**	
B	**F.**	The gland curls around the posterior border of the mylohyoid muscle; this defines the border between its lobes. Hyoglossus lies deep to the gland in the floor of the mouth.
C	**F.**	The duct runs forward and medially from the anterior aspect of the deep lobe, and opens near the midline at the base of the frenulum.
D	**T.**	This nerve, which supplies the corner of the mouth, is at risk during excision of the gland. It can be avoided by placing the incision just above the level of the hyoid and carrying out the dissection in the plane between gland and capsule.
E	**T.**	It runs forward and upward over the superficial lobe.

261

A	**F.**	It lies below the middle cranial fossa.
B	**T.**	It continues down into the neck and superior mediastinum.
C	**T.**	
D	**F.**	Maxillary artery and mandibular nerve.
E	**T.**	The plexus is formed around and within the lateral pterygoid muscle.

262

A	**T.**	
B	**T.**	Hinge movements occur mainly in the lower compartment, sliding in the upper.
C	**F.**	Lateral pterygoid.
D	**T.**	This muscle is inserted into a pit on the anterior border of the mandibular ramus just below the joint, and also into the articular disc.
E	**F.**	Mandibular division, mainly from the auriculotemporal branch.

263 The soft palate

A   The palatine aponeurosis is formed by the expanded tendons of levator palati muscles.

B   Tensor palati turns through 90 degrees around the pterygoid hamulus.

C   Contains mucous glands, lymphoid tissue and taste buds.

D   Is lined by squamous epithelium on its superior surface.

E   Main blood supply comes from the greater palatine artery.

264 Derivatives of the pharyngeal pouches

A   The intratonsillar cleft is a remnant of the second pouch.

B   Parathyroid tissue develops from the fourth and fifth.

C   The ultimobranchial body is a fifth pouch derivative.

D   Branchial cysts usually lie posterior to sternomastoid.

E   The thyroid gland is derived from the fourth pouch.

265 White lesions of the oral cavity

A   Leucoplakia can be rubbed off.

B   Candidiasis may appear as a red or white area.

C   Vitamin B12 deficiency causes white patches on the tongue.

D   A pattern of red areas with white or yellow elevated borders which changes from day to day should be biopsied.

E   Lace-like pattern is characteristic of lichen planus.

263

A   **F.**   Formed by the expanded tendons of tensor palati muscles, which meet in a midline raphe. This is the functional basis of the soft palate. All other muscles except musculus uvulae insert into it.

B   **T.**

C   **T.**

D   **F.**   Upper (nasopharyngeal) surface is lined by respiratory epithelium, lower by non-keratinizing stratified squamous.

E   **F.**   The main blood supply is from the palatine branch of the ascending pharyngeal. The greater palatine artery supplies primarily the hard palate, it runs forward from the greater palatine foramen to the incisive canal.

264

A   **T.**

B   **F.**   Third and fourth, the third being inferior to the fourth in the adult.

C   **T.**   The ultimobranchial body is thought to be the source of the C cells of the thyroid, which produce calcitonin.

D   **F.**   Anterior. There is dispute as to whether branchial cysts are truly of branchial origin. Against the congenital theory is the fact that most do not present until early adult life. A popular alternative theory is that branchial cysts arise from epithelial cell rests within lymph nodes.

E   **F.**   The thyroid gland is derived from the thyroglossal duct. The C cells are from the fifth pouch.

265

A   **F.**   The definition of leucoplakia is a white patch which cannot be rubbed off.

B   **T.**

C   **F.**   Causes a red beefy tongue.

D   **F.**   The description is of geographical tongue. Management consists of reassurance.

E   **T.**   Not always present, the oral lesions may be simple white plaques. There may also be pinkish patches on the skin.

266 Mouth ulcers
A   Aphthous ulcers are not usually painful.
B   Herpes simplex ulceration in children may be complicated by acute encephalitis.
C   Ulcers of the mouth and genitalia with uveitis characterize Reiter's syndrome.
D   Local steroids are used in the treatment of aphthous ulcers.
E   Pemphigus vulgaris should be treated by masterly inactivity.

267 Tumours of the oral cavity
A   An epulis is a midline bony lesion of the hard palate.
B   Papilloma is caused by a DNA virus.
C   Minor salivary gland tumours are almost always benign.
D   A chronic ulcer in the floor of the mouth is likely to be malignant.
E   Carcinoma is commoner on the lower lip than the upper.

268 Salivary gland tumours
A   The commonest parotid tumour is the adenoid cystic carcinoma.
B   The adenolymphoma (Warthin's tumour) is commoner in young women, is painful and grows rapidly.
C   A submandibular tumour is more likely to be malignant than a parotid tumour.
D   In mucoepidermoid carcinoma, recurrence rates and survival correlate with histological grade.
E   Distant metastases after many years are characteristic of adenoid cystic carcinoma.

266

A	**F.**	Pain is the major symptom and can be severe.
B	**T.**	Intravenous acyclovir is used to treat this complication.
C	**F.**	The description is of Behçet's syndrome. Reiter's is characterized by iritis and arthritis following either urethritis or dysentery.
D	**T.**	Either pellets to be sucked, or applied as a paste.
E	**F.**	Likely to be followed by forced inactivity, as the condition is fatal without aggressive steroid treatment!

267

A	**F.**	An epulis is any soft tissue swelling of the gums. The midline bony swelling of the palate is the torus palatinus.
B	**T.**	The human papilloma virus. There are various strains, each with a penchant for certain sites.
C	**F.**	50% are malignant, mainly adenoid cystic carcinoma.
D	**T.**	The so called 'sump areas'.
E	**T.**	Probably because of sunlight exposure. Commoner in outdoor workers.

268

A	**F.**	The commonest is pleomorphic adenoma (mixed parotid tumour) which accounts for 80% of cases.
B	**F.**	85% in males, mostly aged 50–70. Slow growing, painless, bilateral in 10% of cases. They are characteristically soft and may be fluctuant.
C	**T.**	20% of parotid tumours are malignant, 40% of submandibular tumours. However because parotid tumours are much commoner than submandibular (ratio 10 to 1) the overall incidence of malignant parotid tumours is greater than that of malignant submandibular tumours.
D	**T.**	Low grade mucoepidermoid carcinoma recurs locally in 6% of cases and has a 90% 5 year survival rate, whereas high grade recurs in up to 80% and only 20% survive 5 years. In addition, metastasis is rare in low grade tumours but occurs in 60% of high grade.
E	**T.**	Commonest in the lung, may recur up to 20 years after apparently successful removal of the primary.

269 Benign salivary gland disease

A   Calculi occur more commonly in the mucous secreting salivary glands than in the serous.
B   Unilateral parotid gland enlargement may occur in mumps.
C   Mikulicz syndrome consists of bilateral enlargement of the lacrimal, parotid and submandibular glands.
D   Sjögren's syndrome has the same salivary gland changes as Mikulicz syndrome in association with a connective tissue disease, usually rheumatoid arthritis.
E   Malignant lymphoma arising in the affected salivary glands is a recognized complication of Sjögren's syndrome.

270 During deglutition

A   Elevation of the hyoid bone reduces the size of the oral cavity.
B   Passavant's bar assists closure of the nasopharyngeal hiatus.
C   A fixed thyroid cartilage is necessary in the pharyngeal phase.
D   The epiglottis directs the food stream into 2 lateral channels.
E   A peristaltic wave starts in the top of the pharynx as the bolus enters the oesophagus.

269

A **T.** Approximately 80% occur in the submandibular gland, which is mainly mucous. Stones are rare in the parotid, which is mainly serous.

B **T.** Usually bilateral, but can be unilateral. Orchitis, pancreatitis and hepatitis may be associated.

C **T.** Described by Mikulicz in 1888. The term 'benign lymphoepithelial lesion' was proposed by Godwin in 1952 and is now preferred.

D **T.** Described by Sjögren in 1933. Keratoconjunctivitis sicca and xerostomia with enlargement of salivary and lacrimal glands are the main symptoms. It occurs in association with rheumatoid arthritis, polymyositis, systemic lupus erythematosis, scleroderma and polyarteritis nodosa.

E **T.** Occurs in around 5% of cases.

270

A **T.** This ensures that elevation of the tongue from before backwards forces the food bolus posteriorly into the pharynx.

B **T.** Contraction of the laterally placed palatopharyngeal muscles produces this ridge and assists closure by approximating with the elevated soft palate (levator and tensor palatini).

C **F.** Closure of the laryngeal inlet is effected by elevation of the larynx under the shelter of the tongue base. A fixed cartilage would allow aspiration of food. Other factors in closure of the laryngeal isthmus include inhibition of respiration, closure of laryngeal sphincters (aryepiglottic folds, thyro-arytenoid muscles and false cords) and the action of the epiglottis.

D **T.** Toward the pyriform fossae.

E **T.** This wave travels caudally and clears food behind the bolus and also produces contraction of the cricopharyngeus to prevent regurgitation.

271 Pathophysiology of swallowing

A   In bulbar palsy swallowing of liquids is characteristically more difficult than solids.

B   A vagal paralysis has its main clinical effect on the oesophageal phase of swallowing.

C   Cricopharyngeal myotomy is of no benefit if the cause of dysphagia is neurological.

D   Globus pharyngis may be associated with gastro-oesophageal reflux.

E   Tertiary oesophageal contractions occur frequently during emotional stress.

272 Stertor

A   Is defined as noisy respiration due to partial airway obstruction below the level of the epiglottis.

B   The Venturi effect is implicated in causing the noise.

C   The noise is loudest on expiration.

D   Intercostal recession is a feature of severe stertor.

E   Large tonsils and adenoids may be causative.

273 Sleep apnoea in children

A   Is a potential cause of sudden infant death syndrome.

B   Is associated with failure to thrive and feeding difficulties in the infant.

C   Bradycardia is a sign of minor importance.

D   A retropharyngeal swelling is best shown on an occipitomental X-ray.

E   In Pierre–Robin syndrome the respiratory obstruction is most likely to occur in the prone position.

271

A	**T.**	In particular, aspiration is more of a problem.
B	**F.**	The major clinical effect is seen on the pharyngeal phase, especially failure of laryngeal closure leading to aspiration.
C	**F.**	The operation is of benefit in cases where failure of relaxation or spasm are causing symptoms; many of these will be neurological in origin.
D	**T.**	In 15–30% of cases. Antacid medication is frequently effective.
E	**T.**	Tertiary contractions are irregular, non-propulsive contractions involving long segments of the oesophagus. The primary peristaltic wave is that which is initiated by swallowing. Secondary peristaltic waves are initiated by the presence of a bolus within the lumen of the oesophagus.

272

A	**F.**	Partial airway obstruction above the level of the larynx.
B	**T.**	The Venturi effect is the fall in lateral pressure exerted by a gas when it moves along a tube. The fall in pressure is greater if the flow per unit area is increased because of narrowing of the tube. If the walls of the tube are not sufficiently rigid they will collapse inward. The flow then ceases and the pressure drop returns to normal. This cycle, rapidly repeated, causes the noise of stertor.
C	**F.**	Stertor occurs on inspiration. On expiration the intramural pressure is greater than extramural.
D	**T.**	
E	**T.**	Probably the commonest cause.

273

A	**T.**	There are numerous possible causes for this syndrome; certainly sleep apnoea is known to cause sudden infant death.
B	**T.**	
C	**F.**	Bradycardia implies a dangerous degree of hypoxaemia requiring immediate measures to restore an adequate airway.
D	**F.**	Best shown on a soft tissue lateral view.
E	**F.**	Pierre–Robin syndrome is cleft palate and micrognathia. Respiratory obstruction is most likely in the supine position. The position of choice for nursing the affected neonate is prone.

274 Diphtheria
A   Is caused by the *Mycobacterium diphtheriae*, which is a normal commensal of the upper airways in 30% of the UK population.
B   Vaccination is ineffective.
C   An endotoxin is responsible for death by myocarditis.
D   The membrane is easily removed by swabbing.
E   In the suspected case, treatment is deferred pending the results of a Schick test.

275 Chronic non-specific pharyngitis
A   Is associated with smoking.
B   Is exacerbated by chronic bronchitis.
C   Lymphoid hypertrophy is seen in some cases.
D   Treatment with Mandl's paint (applied with a camel hair brush) was last recommended in a major British textbook in 1948.
E   The use of liquid paraffin is no longer recommended because of the risk of lipoid pneumonia.

276 Chronic specific pharyngitis
A   A gumma is a feature of secondary syphilis.
B   Serological tests for syphilis are often negative in the presence of a chancre.
C   Tuberculosis may cause painful pharyngeal ulceration.
D   Scarring does not occur if tuberculosis is treated with antituberculous drugs.
E   Lepromatous ulcers are usually painless.

274
  A **F.**   Caused by *Corynebacterium diphtheriae,* of which
              there are several strains, mitis being least serious and
              gravis most. These are not the same as the
              'Diphtheroid' organisms which are common
              commensals in the upper air and food passages.
  B **F.**   The vaccine is given as part of the 'triple vaccine',
              diphtheria/pertussis/tetanus, to infants at 3,6 and 9
              months. It has been a very successful public health
              measure. Diphtheria is now a rare disease in the UK,
              but cases do occur in unvaccinated patients.
  C **F.**   An exotoxin.
  D **F.**   The membrane is characteristically thick, grey and
              adherent. Removal causes bleeding.
  E **F.**   If the condition is suspected, antitoxin must be given
              urgently because of the risk of sudden death from
              myocarditis or respiratory obstruction. The Schick test
              is a test to determine susceptibility. A purified
              derivative of toxin is injected into the skin and the local
              inflammatory response noted. The test has a role in
              screening contacts after an outbreak to determine
              whether immunization is required.

275
  A **T.**
  B **T.**   Due to the repeated physical trauma of coughing and
              the chronic presence of infected sputum.
  C **T.**   Gives the pharyngeal wall a granular appearance.
  D **F.**   Recommended in Scott-Brown 4th Edn (1979) Vol. 4,
              p. 85.
  E **T.**

276
  A **F.**   A gumma is seen in tertiary syphilis. Snail track ulcers
              (symmetrically placed), mucous patches and rubbery
              cervical lymphadenopathy are the characteristic
              features of secondary syphilis.
  B **T.**   The diagnosis is made by examining a smear taken
              from the lesion under dark ground illumination, when
              the spirochaetes will be seen.
  C **T.**
  D **F.**   Severe scarring with stenosis occurs despite
              treatment.
  E **T.**   Because the peripheral nerve endings are destroyed.

277 Acute tonsillitis
A   Peak incidence is in the age group 1–3 years.
B   A preceding viral infection of the upper respiratory tract
     predisposes.
C   The alpha-haemolytic streptococcus is the commonest
     bacterial cause.
D   Enlargement of the jugulodigastric lymph nodes is rarely seen
     except in glandular fever.
E   In infectious mononucleosis (glandular fever) the absolute
     lymphocyte count is reduced.

278 Quinsy
A   Is defined as a peritonsillar abscess.
B   Is commonest in children.
C   The pus lies in the space between the superior constrictor
     muscle and the carotid sheath.
D   Trismus and dribbling are clinical features.
E   Treatment consists of systemic antibiotics and drainage.

279 Tonsillectomy
A   Indications include central sleep apnoea.
B   A family history of bleeding is an absolute contraindication.
C   The dissection method is quicker than the guillotine.
D   The Boyle–Davis gag with Doughty modification is used with
     nasotracheal intubation.
E   A major arterial bleed can occur from the facial artery.

280 Benign tumours of the oropharynx
A   Commonest is the squamous cell papilloma.
B   A virus is implicated in the aetiology of squamous cell
     papilloma.
C   A smooth swelling of the lateral wall should be biopsied
     transorally.
D   Most tonsillar tumours are benign.
E   Salivary gland tumours rarely occur in the soft palate.

277

A	**F.**	4–6 years.
B	**T.**	
C	**F.**	Beta-haemolytic streptococcus.
D	**F.**	Enlargement of the local nodes is very common.
E	**F.**	There is a lymphocytosis, with the presence of atypical lymphocytes. The Paul–Bunnell test is positive.

278

A	**T.**	
B	**F.**	Commonest in young adults.
C	**F.**	That would be a parapharyngeal abscess, which may complicate a quinsy. In a quinsy, the pus lies in the space between the tonsil and its capsule.
D	**T.**	
E	**T.**	Drainage may be carried out by incision under surface anaesthesia. Quinsy tonsillectomy is an alternative, rarely performed.

279

A	**F.**	Obstructive sleep apnoea.
B	**F.**	An indication for studies of clotting profile.
C	**F.**	But it is more precise and has fewer complications and is therefore preferred.
D	**F.**	The Doughty modification is the split blade for the gag, which is used for orotracheal intubation in children. It is necessary because adenoidectomy, which is often carried out at the same operation, contraindicates the use of a nasal tube.
E	**T.**	It loops just lateral to the superior constrictor and can be damaged during dissection of a fibrotic tonsillar bed, particularly in adults.

280

A	**T.**	
B	**T.**	Human papilloma virus.
C	**F.**	May be a deep lobe parotid tumour, a neurogenous tumour, a paraganglioma or a carotid aneurysm. These will require an external approach following preoperative CT or angiographic evaluation.
D	**F.**	Most are malignant, squamous carcinoma or lymphoma.
E	**T.**	Commoner on the hard palate, which is part of the oral cavity.

281 Malignant tumours of the oropharynx
A   Sites include faucial pillars, soft palate, tonsil, base of tongue, vallecula and posterior pharyngeal wall.
B   The commonest site is the base of tongue.
C   Squamous carcinoma, lymphoma and salivary gland tumours occur in that order of frequency.
D   Lymph node metastases are rare in squamous carcinoma.
E   Full TNM classification requires a CT scan.

282 Lymphoma of the oropharynx
A   Most cases are Hodgkin's.
B   The B-cell is the commonest cell of origin.
C   Burkitt's lymphoma is associated with Herpes simplex virus.
D   Investigations should include exploratory laparotomy.
E   Complete surgical excision is the treatment of choice.

283 Treatment of squamous carcinoma of the tonsil
A   Surgery is of no benefit if there are lymph node metastases.
B   Radiotherapy is only given for palliation.
C   A pectoralis major myocutaneous flap can be used to reconstruct after resection of the primary and radical neck dissection.
D   The general condition of the patient is of major prognostic significance.
E   Cisplatin has been shown to prolong survival in Phase III trials.

281

A	**T.**	In addition, the anterior (lingual) surface of the epiglottis is included in the UICC classification, but in the AJC system it is regarded as part of the larynx.
B	**F.**	Commonest site is the tonsil (50%). Base of tongue tumours account for around 25% of cases.
C	**T.**	70%, 25% and 5%.
D	**F.**	Nodal metastases occur in at least 60% of cases.
E	**F.**	CT scan is optional, endoscopy and histological confirmation are mandatory.

282

A	**F.**	The majority are Non-Hodgkin's of high grade malignancy.
B	**T.**	
C	**F.**	Epstein–Barr virus.
D	**F.**	Not necessary with modern radiological techniques, e.g. abdominal CT scanning.
E	**F.**	Unlikely to be achieved. These tumours are particularly sensitive to radiotherapy and chemotherapy and combinations of the two are the treatment of choice.

283

A	**F.**	Radical neck dissection is the best available treatment for neck node metastases, provided they are unilateral, not fixed, and less than 6 cm diameter. It can be carried out in continuity with removal of the primary in a COMMANDO operation (COMbined neck dissection, MANDibulectomy and resection of Oropharynx).
B	**F.**	Cure can be achieved with radiotherapy alone in favourable cases, i.e. small tumour, no nodes, patient's general condition good. Radiotherapy is also used in combination with surgical excision in planned combined treatment, which gives 5 year survival rates of the order of 30%.
C	**T.**	The commonest method today, although microvascular free flaps are increasingly used for reconstruction in head and neck surgery.
D	**T.**	
E	**T.**	By a median 3 months. Unfortunately this is well short of cure.

284 Hypopharyngeal tumours
A   Sites include pyriform fossa, postcricoid region and vallecula.
B   Benign tumours are common.
C   Postcricoid carcinoma is commoner in women.
D   Pyriform fossa tumours spread laterally into the paraglottic space.
E   A T3 tumour is associated with a fixed vocal cord and means that the recurrent laryngeal nerve has been invaded.

285 Carcinoma of the pyriform fossa
A   Is commonest in males aged 50–70 years.
B   Dysphagia with pain on swallowing radiating to the ear is characteristic.
C   Presentation as a neck node with 'unknown primary' is not uncommon.
D   Occult nodal metastases are present in over 30% of clinically non-palpable necks.
E   Surgical treatment usually allows preservation of the larynx.

286 Total pharyngolaryngectomy
A   The main indication is squamous carcinoma of the postcricoid region.
B   Primary anastamosis of the orostome to the cervical oesophagus is achieved in the majority of cases.
C   The thyroid gland is removed.
D   The pectoralis major myocutaneous flap can be used for reconstruction.
E   The free jejunal graft with microvascular anastamosis is only suitable for disease confined to the neck.

284

A **F.** The hypopharynx (UICC definition) extends from the level of the hyoid bone to the lower border of the cricoid cartilage. The vallecula is part of the oropharynx. The third hypopharyngeal site is the posterior pharyngeal wall, between the level of the floor of the vallecula and the cricoarytenoid joints.

B **F.** 99% are malignant, nearly all squamous carcinoma.

C **T.** Ratio 2:1.

D **F.** The paraglottic space is medial to the pyriform fossa. Lateral spread is via the thyrohyoid membrane.

E **F.** There is fixation, but this can be due to invasion of muscles or cricoarytenoid joint as well as recurrent laryngeal nerve involvement.

285

A **T.**

B **T.**

C **T.**

D **T.**

E **F.** Total laryngectomy is required because the larynx is nearly always invaded via the paraglottic space. Also, if there is an insufficient margin of uninvolved pharyngeal mucosa to allow primary closure of an adequate food passage, a total laryngopharyngectomy with pharyngeal reconstruction will be required.

286

A **T.** Also indicated for extensive pyriform fossa carcinoma lesions and upper oesophageal tumours.

B **F.** This manoeuvre is not a practical surgical option because of the segmental blood supply of the oesophagus. In addition there is frequently extensive submucosal spread of disease in the oesophagus so oesophagectomy is desirable on oncological grounds.

C **T.**

D **T.**

E **T.**

287 Total pharyngolaryngectomy and oesophagectomy
  A   Gastric transposition necessitates cervical, thoracic and
        abdominal incisions.
  B   Colon transposition has the disadvantage of three
        anastamoses.
  C   Stenosis is the main complication of using stomach for the
        repair.
  D   Postoperative thyroid and calcium supplements are required.
  E   A pneumothorax is treated by insertion of a chest drain.

288 Recurrence of hypopharyngeal carcinoma
  A   Distant metastases are the usual cause of death.
  B   Regular follow-up examination provides reliable early detection.
  C   Possible causes include tumour implantation at operation.
  D   Stomal recurrence can be treated by thoracotracheostomy with
        manubrial resection, but is rarely successful.
  E   May present as a persistent pharyngocutaneous fistula.

289 Malignant cervical lymph nodes
  A   Assessment for TNM staging by palpation is subject to inter-
        observer variation of around 30% among trained specialists.
  B   Palpable nodes not infrequently contain no tumour.
  C   Non-palpable nodes not infrequently contain tumour.
  D   Nodes in the supraclavicular fossa carry a worse prognosis
        than nodes in the submandibular triangle.
  E   Because of the unreliability of assessment, N-status is
        unrelated to prognosis.

287

A **F.** Thoracic incision is not necessary, the thoracic oesophagus can be freed by blind finger dissection from below and the mobilized stomach can be passed up in a similar way. However there is a risk of massive haemorrhage and the surgical team must be prepared to do an immediate thoracotomy if required.

B **T.** One in the neck, one between lower end of transposed colon and stomach, and one to restore continuity between ileum and descending colon (the caecum and terminal ileum are discarded).

C **F.** Stenosis is very rare. The main complication is the operative mortality (5–25%).

D **T.** Because the thyroid and parathyroids are removed.

E **T.** An underwater seal chest drain.

288

A **F.** Loco-regional recurrence, at the primary site, resection margins and cervical nodes, is the commonest.

B **F.** Early detection is difficult because of the radiotherapy reaction and scarring which follows earlier therapy.

C **T.**

D **T.**

E **T.**

289

A **T.**

B **T.** Only 60% of palpable nodes contained tumour in one study.

C **T.** Depending on site and T stage of primary. In oropharyngeal, hypopharyngeal and supraglottic laryngeal primaries (T2 and greater) there is a high risk of occult nodal metastases.

D **T.**

E **F.** N-status correlates well with prognosis; there is little difficulty with classifying patients who have large, fixed or bilateral nodes and these have a very poor prognosis.

290 Radical neck dissection
A   Consists of removal of all the lymph-bearing structures between the midline, mandible, anterior border of sternomastoid and clavicle.
B   The sternomastoid muscle, internal jugular vein, and submandibular gland are excised with the specimen.
C   The upper end of the internal jugular vein is divided first.
D   The accessory nerve is preserved.
E   A chylous leak during a left-sided operation is recognized as milky fluid collecting in the lower part of the wound.

291 Functional neck dissection
A   Aims to remove only nodes and tissue likely to be involved by tumour.
B   Published indications include the clinically NO neck with high risk of occult metastases.
C   Papillary carcinoma of the thyroid is a generally accepted indication.
D   The accessory nerve is preserved.
E   Crile never performed such a procedure.

292 Pharyngeal pouch (Zenker's diverticulum)
A   Origin is between middle and inferior constrictor muscles (Dehiscence of Killian).
B   The cause is traction by contracting tuberculous scar tissue.
C   Associated symptoms include dysphagia and dyspnoea.
D   Dohlman's operation is an endoscopic excision of the pouch.
E   Inversion of the pouch is an alternative to excision.

290
A **F.** Anterior border of trapezius. The area described is the anterior triangle only.
B **T.**
C **F.** The lower end, to prevent tumour embolization during subsequent dissection.
D **F.** It is divided at the anterior border of trapezius.
E **F.** The patient will have been starved, so the chyle is clear.

291
A **T.** The risk is that unrecognized tumour will be left behind.
B **T.** The argument against elective neck dissection in general is that survival is not improved compared with a 'wait and see' policy, with surgery for recurrences.
C **T.**
D **T.** Plus or minus the sternomastoid, internal jugular vein, cervical plexus and submandibular gland.
E **F.** Crile preserved jugular vein and sternomastoid in cases without palpable nodes.

292
A **F.** The dehiscence is between the two parts of inferior constrictor, thyropharyngeus and cricopharyngeus.
B **F.** It is a pulsion diverticulum, raised intrapharyngeal pressure causes bulging of mucosa through the weak zone posteriorly. There is failure of normal coordination of swallowing, but the underlying cause of this is not known.
C **T.** Dysphagia is an early symptom, dyspnoea comes later because of aspiration pneumonia.
D **F.** Endoscopic diathermy division of the party wall between diverticulum and oesophagus. Special instruments are required.
E **T.** Easier, less risk of infection since the pharynx is not opened, less risk of stricture and less risk of damaging the recurrent laryngeal nerve. There is a small risk of developing a carcinoma on the inverted sac mucosa.

293 Thyroglossal cysts and sinuses
A   Result from developmental abnormalities of the descent of the thyroid from the foramen caecum.
B   Usually present as a midline neck swelling in a child or young adult.
C   The majority are above the level of the hyoid.
D   An infected cyst should be incised and drained.
E   In Sistrunk's operation, the entire hyoid bone is removed.

294 Branchial sinuses and fistulae
A   The majority are present at birth.
B   Internal opening in the supratonsillar fossa implies origin from the cervical sinus of His.
C   A tract passing between internal and external carotid arteries suggests origin from the first branchial cleft.
D   A collaural fistula has two openings.
E   First line treatment consists of injection of sclerosants.

295 Branchial cysts
A   Most are associated with internal openings.
B   Histology supports the theory of origin from squamous cell rests within lymph nodes.
C   Peak age of onset is 20–30 years.
D   Aspiration should never be performed because of the risk of implanting cholesterol crystals in the neck.
E   Hodgkin's disease is part of the differential diagnosis.

293

A	**T.**	
B	**T.**	90% are midline. 66% in patients under 30. The lump moves up on protruding the tongue and on swallowing.
C	**F.**	Only 25% are suprahyoid.
D	**F.**	Makes subsequent excision difficult. Should be treated with antibiotics, with definitive excision as an elective procedure. Needle aspiration is a useful method for dealing with the acute episode, but if the contents are very viscid may not be possible.
E	**F.**	Only the body of the hyoid is removed.

294

A	**T.**	Unlike branchial cysts which usually present in early adult life.
B	**F.**	Implies origin from the second pharyngeal pouch. The cervical sinus is formed by a ventral overgrowth of the second arch, which comes to overlie the remaining arches and clefts caudal to it. It fuses with the neck skin (C2) burying the ectoderm of the third, fourth and sixth arches. There is normally no communication with the lumen of the pharynx.
C	**F.**	Second pouch. First branchial pouch abnormalities may account for cysts high in the neck and fistulae opening in the external auditory meatus.
D	**T.**	Any true fistula has two openings. The collaural fistula passes between the external auditory meatus and the skin of the neck, opening between angle of mandible and sternomastoid. It is probably a first cleft defect.
E	**F.**	Treatment, if required, is excision of the whole tract.

295

A	**F.**	A rare occurrence.
B	**T.**	Most are lined with squamous epithelium and have lymphoid tissue in their walls.
C	**T.**	
D	**F.**	Nonsense.
E	**T.**	Also other lymphomas, secondary deposits, paraganglioma, tuberculosis, and reactive lymphadenitis.

296 In the oesophagus
A   The pharynx joins it at the glossoepiglottic folds.
B   There are only 2 constrictions along its length.
C   The non-striated muscle has a motor supply from the vagus.
D   Portal-systemic anastamoses are located in the middle third.
E   The cricopharyngeal sphincter is about 3 cm in length.

297 The lower oesophageal sphincter
A   Can be demonstrated histologically.
B   A pinch cock effect is produced by the left crus of the diaphragm.
C   May be merely mucosal folds in the lower end of the oesophagus.
D   A normal oesophagogastric angle prevents acid reflux.
E   The sling of Willis is essential in sphincteric action.

298 Congenital oesophageal atresia
A   Over 80% of cases are associated with a tracheo-oesophageal fistula.
B   Gas in the gastro-intestinal tract implies the presence of polyhydramnios.
C   Feeding may produce aspiration pneumonitis.
D   After successful surgical correction swallowing develops normally.
E   Mortality is related to the site of the defect.

296

A **F.**   The oesophagus starts and the pharynx ends at the lower border of the cricoid cartilage. In the adult at the level of the 6th cervical vertebra.

B **F.**   There are 3. Each one may be a site of impaction of a foreign body. From the incisor teeth they are; at 15 cm the cricopharyngeal sphincter; at 25 cm where the aortic arch and left main bronchus cross the oesophagus and at 40 cm the region of the gastro-oesophageal sphincter.

C **T.**   In the lower two thirds. It is mainly parasympathetic and the cell bodies are in the vagal nucleus. The upper third is striated and supplied by the recurrent nerves.

D **F.**   Located in the lower third and can produce varices secondary to portal obstruction with a potential risk of haemorrhage.

E **T.**   The middle 1 cm zone shows the greatest rise in pressure on manometry.

297

A **F.**   There is no thickening of the circular muscle layer. Therefore called a 'physiological' sphincter.

B **F.**   By the right crus as it splits to encircle the oesophagus.

C **T.**   The folds may have a valvular effect.

D **F.**   Can occur despite a normal angle. However, the sharp angle may act as a mechanical flap valve.

E **F.**   The sling is the oblique muscle fibres of the stomach encircling the lower oesophagus. However, this site does not correspond to the sphincteric mechanism and the anti reflux mechanism is still present after section of the sling fibres.

298

A **T.**   The majority will be distal fistulae. In the neonate these can lead to aspiration of meconium.

B **F.**   Gas in the gastrointestinal tract below the atresia indicates the presence of a tracheo-oesophageal fistula. Polyhydramnios occurs in 30% of mothers due to the inability of the foetus to swallow amniotic fluid.

C **T.**   Either by overspill into trachea or via a tracheo-oesophageal fistula. If atresia is suspected the first feed should be withheld.

D **F.**   Difficulties may persist for years due to stricture or oesophageal dysmobility.

E **F.**   Dependent on associated abnormalities particularly cardiac defects.

299 Hiatus hernia
  A   A para-oesophageal hernia is more likely to produce reflux than a sliding hernia.
  B   Dysphagia is the most commonly presenting complaint.
  C   A gastric air shadow is seen in the sliding variety.
  D   Surgery is particularly indicated in para-oesophageal herniae.
  E   Recurrence rate after surgery is about 10–15%.

300 Perforation of the oesophagus
  A   Is more likely to occur with a flexible than rigid oesophagoscope.
  B   Severe vomiting may produce a tear in the middle third.
  C   Cervical surgical emphysema can always be elicited.
  D   If treatment is delayed more than 24 h the mortality is about 50%.
  E   Contrast X-ray studies should not be performed.

301 Clinical features of a foreign body in the oesophagus include
  A   Back pain.
  B   Hoarseness.
  C   Dyspnoea.
  D   Absence of laryngeal crepitus.
  E   Excessive salivation.

299

A **F.** The reverse is true. In the para-oesophageal hernia the gastro-oesophageal function is retained below the diaphragm but a portion of the stomach protrudes through the hiatus. Mixed herniae can occur.

B **F.** The commonest symptoms are heartburn and retrosternal discomfort.

C **F.** Seen in the para-oesophageal type on a lateral chest X-ray and is located posterior to the heart.

D **T.** To prevent complications such as anaemia, pseudo angina (obstruction or impaction).

E **T.** But the symptoms are usually ameliorated and may be more readily controlled with medical treatment.

300

A **F.** The former has reduced the incidence of perforation due to instrumentation.

B **F.** Most frequently the lower end. A longitudinal tear involving all layers of the viscus.

C **F.** If the thoracic oesophagus is involved this sign may be absent. Air under the diaphragm may be present in ruptures of the abdominal portion.

D **T.** Early diagnosed cervical tears may be managed conservatively but thoracic tears rarely respond to medical treatment. Surgery for repair and or drainage should not be delayed if the clinical picture demands it.

E **F.** May delineate site and aetiology of perforation. Dionysil opaque medium should be used.

301

A **T.** Pain referred to the back or retrosternum, particularly if the foreign object is in the middle or lower third oesophagus and therefore poorly localized.

B **T.** Impaction at the cricopharyngeal sphincter may lead to laryngeal oedema.

C **T.** Same reason as (b) and in children because the trachea may be compressed by the foreign object.

D **T.** Due to oesophageal oedema. Localized tenderness is present on laryngeal palpation.

E **T.** As saliva pools in the pyriform fossae.

302 Benign neoplasms of the oesophagus
A   Account for about 25% of oesophageal neoplasms.
B   Smooth muscle tumours are the most common.
C   May be regurgitated into the mouth.
D   Leiomyomas are readily visualized during endoscopy.
E   Dysphagia is uncommon.

303 Carcinoma of the oesophagus
A   A very high incidence occurs in Bantu tribesmen.
B   Tends to develop at sites of normal narrowing.
C   May develop in achalasia.
D   Cigarette smoking is not a risk factor.
E   Is more common in females.

304 Management of oesophageal cancer
A   The right colon is the most suitable portion of the colon for interposition.
B   The argon laser is a useful tool for vaporization of tumour.
C   The Mousseau Barbin tube is pushed through a tumour stricture.
D   Radiotherapy is likely to produce radiation corditis.
E   Gastrostomy is essential to maintain nutrition after resection.

305 Oesophageal stricture
A   Is most commonly due to reflux oesophagitis.
B   Endoscopy is not required if barium studies reveal a smooth narrowing.
C   Shatski's ring can cause narrowing.
D   May be caused by ingesting potassium salts.
E   Peptic reflux strictures should be bougienaged if causing dysphagia.

302

A	**F.**	Less than 10% are benign.
B	**T.**	Accounting for about 60% of all benign tumours.
C	**T.**	Particularly if they are pedunculated and located in the upper oesophagus.
D	**F.**	As they are submucosal and easily missed.
E	**T.**	Main symptom is the feeling of a lump in the throat, only latterly producing dysphagia.

303

A	**T.**	Probably due to ingestion of nitrosamine carcinogens from cooking pots.
B	**T.**	Particularly the junction of the pharyngo-oesophagus and where the aorta and left main bronchus crosses it.
C	**T.**	Even in patients who have previously been treated.
D	**F.**	It is along with high alcohol consumption.
E	**F.**	Over 75% are male.

304

A	**F.**	The right side is bulky and it has a tenuous blood supply at the ileocaecal region. The left colon is preferred due to less bulk, comparable calibre and its ability to propel solid material. Microvascular free jejunal grafts may be employed for high resections.
B	**F.**	The neodymium YAG is employed as it passes down a flexible tube. Particularly useful for recurrences at anastamotic sites and high lesions.
C	**F.**	It is pulled through the tumour via a gastrostomy.
D	**F.**	Radiation pneumonitis and post-radiation stricture may occur. Radiotherapy is usually palliative if surgery is not contemplated.
E	**F.**	Nasogastric or parenteral feeding allow the anastamosis time to heal. Gastrostomy as a form of palliation is not justified.

305

A	**T.**	
B	**F.**	All cases should have endoscopy to exclude a neoplasm and to assess the precise level and severity of the lesion.
C	**T.**	This is a lower oesophageal web similar to the cervical web at the pharyngo-oesophageal junction (Paterson–Brown–Kelly or Plummer–Vinson syndrome).
D	**T.**	Potassium in diuretic preparations may cause oesophagitis with subsequent narrowing.
E	**T.**	Combined with intensive medical treatment to neutralize acid.

306 Achalasia of the cardia
A   There is abnormal peristalsis in the lower oesophagus.
B   Meissner's ganglion cells in the oesophagus are absent.
C   Amyl nitrate inhalation is the treatment of choice.
D   Ramstedt's operation relieves symptoms in the majority of
     patients.
E   Oesophagectasia may be present.

306

A	**F.**	Peristalsis is absent.
B	**F.**	There is an absence or reduction in cells in Auerbach's plexus.
C	**F.**	May improve swallowing before meals but surgical treatment is favoured.
D	**F.**	Ramstedt's is a myotomy for infantile pyloric stenosis. Heller's operation, which is also a myotomy, is employed in achalasia with excellent symptomatic relief.
E	**T.**	Achalasia and oesophagectasia are synonyms.

SECTION 5
GENERAL AND
RELATED

307 Radiotherapy
A   Cobalt (^{60}Co) produces gamma radiation.
B   Mega voltage beams produce marked skin reactions.
C   Bone necrosis is more likely if total dose delivered is by low voltage beams.
D   Electron absorption is directly proportional to their energy levels.
E   X-rays are a form of piezo-electric radiation.

308 Efficacy of radiotherapy
A   Squamous cell tumours are more responsive than tumours of lymphoid origin.
B   Sarcomata of bony origin have a very poor response rate.
C   Is enhanced by hypothermia.
D   Photons damage cells more effectively than neutrons.
E   Hypoxia protects tumour cells.

309 During a course of radical radiotherapy for head and neck cancer
A   Endarteritis in blood vessels may induce bony necrosis of the maxilla.
B   Radiation mucositis is a sign that the limit of tissue tolerance has been reached.
C   The commonest infection in the oral cavity is aspergillus fumigatis.
D   Wet shaving is essential to remove hair growth that impairs therapy.
E   A rest period is essential every 5 days.

307

A **T.**   Disadvantage of ^{60}Co is that it decays and requires to be replaced every 3–5 years.

B **F.**   They are skin sparing as the maximum dose is delivered deep to the skin. Low voltage beams are useful for superficial skin tumours.

C **T.**   As bone has low transmission and high absorption rates. However, mega voltage beams allow satisfactory tissue absorption and minimize bone absorption.

D **T.**   They have a finite absorption depth and are therefore useful in treating superficial lesions or a block of tissue of known dimensions.

E **F.**   A type of electromagnetic radiation.

308

A **F.**   The reverse is true. Anaplastic and embryonal tumours also have a high response rate but recurrence rates are significant.

B **T.**

C **F.**   Hyperthermia enhances the response to radiotherapy but it is difficult to achieve a temperature difference between tumour and surrounding normal tissue.

D **F.**   Neutrons are more destructive as they are highly charged and densely ionizing. However, the therapeutic ratio is almost one and hence normal tissue is frequently damaged.

E **T.**   Hence the use of hyperbaric oxygen chambers to enhance the effect of radiotherapy. However normal tissue also becomes more richly oxygenated with increased risk of necrosis.

309

A **T.**   It is a particular problem in the mandible.

B **T.**   Trauma, alcohol, tobacco should be avoided, as this enhances the problem. Pain is an associated feature.

C **F.**   Candida albicans is most common. Treatment is by continuous local antifungal therapy in the form of nystatin lozenges or other appropriate preparation.

D **F.**   An electric shaver should be employed to avoid excessive trauma to the skin.

E **F.**   Rest periods should be avoided as the efficacy of the treatment is undermined but may be required if severe reactions occur.

310 Cytotoxic agents in head and neck cancer
A   Cell destruction follows first order kinetics.
B   Cycle specific drugs destroy both resting and cycling cells equally.
C   Methotrexate is a phase specific agent.
D   Synchronization means all cells passing in phase through the cell cycle.
E   Folic acid acts by enhancing the therapeutic effect of methotrexate.

311 Adjuvant chemotherapy in head and neck cancer
A   Impaired renal function precludes the use of methotrexate.
B   A combination of class III anti tumour drugs can be given in normal doses.
C   Pulmonary fibrosis develops in 10% of patients on bleomycin.
D   Cisplatin has a cumulative toxic side effect.
E   The term 'No response' indicates a reduction between 50 and 70% in the product of the 2 largest perpendicular diameters of measurable tumour.

312 Use of lasers in surgery
A   A laser beam is collimated.
B   Thermal effects include contraction of collagen.
C   Vaporization is produced by boiling of intracellular water.
D   A pulsed Nd-YAG laser can produce photomechanical destruction of renal stones.
E   At low power may produce biostimulation.

310

A	**T.**	A given drug dose killing a constant fraction of cells, regardless of the total number of tumour cells present.
B	**F.**	The latter are more sensitive. Cyclophosphamide is an example.
C	**T.**	It destroys proliferating cells during a specific part of the cell cycle.
D	**T.**	
E	**F.**	It reverses the toxic side effects. Employed as 'rescue' therapy for the bone marrow after giving a deliberate overdose of methotrexate. Unfortunately the tumour may also be rescued.

311

A	**F.**	The folinic acid rescue can be extended in such cases.
B	**F.**	Class III combinations should be given in proportionately reduced doses as normal bone marrow stem cells are killed by increasing dosages.
C	**F.**	Only about 1%. However, 10% develop a non-specific pneumonitis.
D	**T.**	These are reduced by adequate prehydration and maintaining a diuresis. Major side effects include nephrotoxicity, ototoxicity and haematological.
E	**F.**	Indicates either no change in size or less than a 50% reduction of measurable tumour.

312

A	**T.**	That is parallel. It is also monochromatic, of a single wavelength and in phase.
B	**T.**	If the tissue temperature rises above 60 ° protein is denatured and this produces contraction. This effect accounts for the haemostatic properties of laser light.
C	**T.**	
D	**T.**	Also gallstones and opaque bodies in the eye.
E	**T.**	Can enhance wound healing.

313 The carbon dioxide laser
   A   Light is absorbed by water.
   B   Can seal blood vessels up to 1 mm in diameter.
   C   Nerve endings are sealed.
   D   Skin incisions heal with greater rapidity.
   E   The light beam can be transmitted by flexible fibres.

314 For the safe use of lasers
   A   The British Standards Code BS 4803 should be complied with.
   B   Metal plating of flexible anaesthetic tubes prevent the possibility of ignition.
   C   Plain glass spectacles will protect the eye from CO_2 laser light.
   D   A laser safety officer should be appointed.
   E   Protective clothing is essential to avoid skin injury.

315 Clinical application of a CO_2 laser
   A   It produces a greater remission rate than interferon in cases of recurrent respiratory papillomatosis.
   B   It reduces recurrence rates when used in removal of intubation granuloma.
   C   Small fenestra can be made in stapedectomy.
   D   Can be employed in the treatment for rhinophyma.
   E   Division of thick vocal cord webs is very successful.

313

A **T.** Since most soft tissues contain between 75 and 90% water light absorption induces boiling and rapid increase in volume.

B **F.** Only up to 0.5 mm in diameter. By defocusing the beam slightly larger vessels can be sealed. The argon laser is more effective in coagulating blood vessels hence its use in ophthalmological vascular pathologies.

C **T.** This may account for the reduction in pain after CO_2 laser surgery. Lymphatics are also sealed with a reduced risk of spread of malignant cells.

D **F.** Skin incisions heal more slowly and initially are of poorer tensile strength.

E **F.** Not the CO_2 laser. The neodymium YAG beam can be transmitted by fibreoptic cable.

314

A **T.**

B **F.** May still ignite if surrounded by oxygen and nitrous oxide. The metal coating may not completely cover the plastic or cracks can appear in it.

C **F.** The spectacles have to attenuate the laser beam to below the maximum permissible exposure. The patient's eyes can be protected with pads soaked in water, eye shields or steel contact lenses.

D **T.** Usually a medical physicist.

E **F.** Unless a direct beam strikes the skin the damage is insignificant.

315

A **F.** Interferon produces excellent regression but with rapid recurrence when treatment is withdrawn.

B **F.**

C **F.** The CO_2 laser has only been used in experimental stapedectomy. The argon laser has been employed in humans but audiometric end results show no difference.

D **T.** Precise dermabrasion is possible.

E **F.** These are usually post traumatic lesions and the recurrence rate is high. Keels are required to prevent recurrence.

316 Photodynamic therapy
A   The phthalocyanines are the most widely used tumour
     sensitizers.
B   Destruction of tissue is by the cytotoxic effect of triplet oxygen.
C   Skin photosensitization lasts up to 8 weeks.
D   HPD is activated at 630 nm wavelength selective.
E   Retention of sensitizer is related to its ingestion by malignant
     cells.

317 Local anaesthetic and vasoconstrictor agents used in ENT
A   Cocaine may cause a rise in blood pressure.
B   The maximum permitted dose of adrenaline is 0.5 ml of 1:1000
     solution.
C   A low pH in tissue will render local anaesthesia less effective.
D   Felypressin has a greater effect on the myocardium than
     adrenaline.
E   If adrenaline is contraindicated prilocaine may be employed.

318 Biomaterials in otolaryngology
A   A biotolerant material does not produce a foreign body
     reaction.
B   Plastipore and proplast are porous alloplasts.
C   Ceravital is a bioactive glass ceramic.
D   Calcium phosphate ceramics have high tensile strength.
E   Cobalt–chromium alloys are corrosion resistant.

316

   A **F.**   Haematoporphyrin derivative (HPD) is. However the tumour to normal tissue take up ratio is low. Experimentally the phthalocyanines have a much higher ratio and may prove to be ideal sensitizers.

   B **F.**   Cytotoxic Singlet oxygen is produced after activation of HPD.

   C **F.**   Usually 3–4 weeks.

   D **T.**   This allows a depth of penetration of 1 cm. HPD is best activated by UV light but the depth of penetration is poor.

   E **F.**   The abnormal tumour circulation retains the sensitizer. The cells do not take up tumour sensitizer.

317

   A **T.**   Dramatic if hypersensitivity is present. Also a falling pulse rate and possible convulsions. But it is a strong vasoconstrictor.

   B **T.**   That is about 100 ml of the standard 1:200 000 solution.

   C **T.**   Acid pH (e.g. in pus and inflamed tissue) increases the ionized particles in the drug and inactivates it.

   D **F.**   Has much lower systemic effects. However, it takes longer to produce vasoconstrictor effects.

   E **T.**   It is less toxic. High doses may produce cyanosis due to methaemoglobin formation.

318

   A **F.**   There is an initial reaction which ceases after incorporation.

   B **T.**   Gained popularity in middle ear reconstruction but the extrusion rate is high.

   C **T.**   Allows bonding between implant and living tissue. Some degradation takes place. Can be difficult to shape when employed in the middle ear.

   D **F.**   Are very brittle. Hydroxyapatite and B Whitlockite have been employed in otology. The former is more biodegradable and may not be replaced by new bone as quickly as it disappears.

   E **T.**   Used in mandibular reconstruction.